Praise For Victoria Teague &
Finding Heaven in the Midst of Hormonal Hell

"In the voice of an experienced counselor and caring friend, Victoria Teague shares a wealth of practical information about the psychological and physiological changes that occur during menopause. Encouraging you each step of the way, often making you laugh, Victoria helps you face the challenges and embrace this season as a time to define what's important, nurture yourself, and pursue lifelong passions."

Pamela Bruner
CEO, Make Your Success Real
Author, Tapping into Ultimate Success

"In *Finding Heaven*, Victoria Teague offers women going through the natural process of peri-menopause and menopause insights and helpful tips that can really make a difference. Victoria's voice helps women understand the diversity of experiences that women can have as they go through this tough time. She also offers support and encouragement as well as clarity for women to be empowered. Thank you, Victoria, for bringing more light to this period in a woman's life that can feel dark at times."

Dr. Zoe Wells
Licensed Naturopathic Doctor
Author, Women's Transformational Journey:
5 Steps to Creating Joy and Balance in Perimenpause

"Once again Victoria Teague has used her masterful storytelling to highlight and affirm women's stories to demonstrate the gift Christ's love is in our lives. This is an uplifting read that will speak to many women as they navigate the changes time brings to us all. I recommend this book to all women seeking to make sense of their 'new normal'."

Welyne M. Thomas, Ph.D.
Partner, IPC

"As menopause begins, there are no alerts. Women may feel as if their body is breaking down, one of their body systems is in jeopardy or their mental capacity is fiercely compromised (feeling they are "going crazy"). It is through the very words of Victoria in this book that women will not only find help, but can totally skip the whole insecurity, mind challenging stage. Victoria's honesty, research and resourcefulness with all of the women that have sought her help is compiled page after page for the benefit of others. I recommend this book for all women, husbands, doctors and counselors. Thank you, Victoria, for your perseverance, research and willingness to fill these pages. You are resourcing more people than you know."

Dr. Sandy Schremmer, D.C., MA
Doctor of Chiropractic & Christian Counselor

"Full of insights and tools, I trust this will be a valuable resource for women during a challenging time. Victoria's courage and honesty are inspiring, and she guides you to not just survive, but ultimately thrive."

Brad Yates
Bestselling Author & YouTube Sensation

"Menopause is a conundrum for physicians because they don't know what to do with it. Chest pain? That they can handle. All hands on deck for chest pain! Menopause? Not so much. As a nurse, I know that women need to be encouraged to tell their stories in order to heal. In this book, Victoria shows us her path through perimenopause and menopause, helping to blaze a trail for others who will follow. I recommend this book! "

Karen Creamer, RN
Author & Holistic Health Coach

"Deals with a sometimes-difficult transition in every woman's life with both humor and moving anecdotes. A heartwarming read."

Bernique Hollis
Mom & Educator

Finding Heaven in the Midst of Hormonal Hell

7 Ways to Breeze through Menopause

Victoria M. Teague

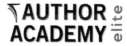

Printed in the United States of America

Published by Author Academy Elite
P.O. Box 43, Powell, OH 43035

www.AuthorAcademyElite.com

Paperback: ISBN 978-1-64085-329-4

Hardback: ISBN 978-1-64085-330-0

Ebook: ISBN 978-1-64085-331-7

Library of Congress Control Number (LCCN): 2018906963

Acknowledgements

I am so grateful that we all operate with many gifts and talents.

This writing project exists because of the encouragement and collaborative work of a special tribe called Author Academy Elite and Kary Oberbrunner. Also, a big thank you to Sallie Boyles, my dear friend and editor. So grateful and thankful for the many hands that helped to bring this project to fruition. I am especially thankful for the team spirit and emotional support that has carried me. Thank YOU, AAE Tribe, from the bottom of my heart.

And a very special thanks to my husband Jeff Teague, who weathered the "hormonal storm" with me well! My love and blessings to all of you!

This Book is dedicated to

Dr. Zoe Wells N.D.
And
Dr. Christiane Northrup M.D.,

the two professionals who made sense out of my "hormonal hell."

Ladies, you are both pioneers who have gone before us to help us make the journey well.

MEDICAL DISCLAIMER

Thank You for Purchasing this Book!
Please Accept My FREE GIFT: 19 Ways to Improve Your Relationships

Increase your passion. Gain and establish trust.
Enjoy the love you've always wanted.
GO TO FindingHeavenBook.com/pages/bonus

Contents

Finding Heaven in the Midst of Hormonal Hell

"A grown woman should not have to masquerade as
a girl in order to remain in the land of the living."
Germaine Greer

A horrible dread came over me. I was topping the hill on a
route I'd driven so many times. My head was swimming
and I was trying to concentrate on the road. Inexplicably, a
fog had kicked in and I could barely see where I was going.
Whether by chance or by fate, the visible fog represented the
state of my mind. I was trying to stay the course and see the
path ahead. I had to reach my children.

Magically, it seemed, the clouds parted. The sky appeared,
and I could see the road. As I looked at the setting sun, a
single goose flew by. His squawking troubled me. It was as if
he were lost and searching. Where's your family, little goose, I
wondered. Did you drop out of the V-formation of your tribe?
Back and forth across my frame of vision, the goose traveled

while squealing in that strange tone. My heart broke for the little fellow. Using my car as his beacon, he followed me around the long bend that led to the lake. When we approached a cove, the goose saw and heard the familiar sounds of his plump (his group of fellow travelers), and he flew toward the sun.

As my brief companion, the goose gave me great comfort; I was not alone. Nevertheless, I felt like a lost bird. At some point I had lost myself. What happened to the self-confident, strong-minded, mover and shaker who was the top sales rep in her corporate gig? Where was the woman who birthed two amazing children while birthing a charity for destitute women? Where did she go?

One day, I was the woman I'd always been. The next, I couldn't think straight. Simple tasks had become drudgery. All I wanted to do was eat and cry! No! Was this menopause?

Yes, my dear, it is the big pause that you're supposed to keep to yourself. Your family is tired of hearing about it. Your doctor has no real answers even though researchers are seeking solutions for women over fifty—a significant and growing percentage of the population. In truth, there's no quick fix. Each one of us is quite different with an individual chemistry.

You, like I, was probably caught off guard as you stumbled into this menopausal season. When younger and thinking ahead, I knew I would soar right through it. After all, I'd made it through every prior season in life with flying colors! Perimenopause, however, wreaked havoc with my diet, my workout, my energy levels, my sex life and my self-esteem. Time after time, a deep fog would come over me, leaving me to shrink back and somehow behave and feel less like the beautiful, strong, independent woman, mother and wife I had become. Yet, I'm here to tell you that I have made this transition and I have great news: There's life—a great life—right on the other side. Yes, you, too, can find heaven in the midst of hormonal hell!

Hero Story

My Aunt Lorene lived to age ninety-one. A graceful and beautiful lady, she truly missed her calling as a model. Along with her beauty, Aunt Lorene had poise, and she was just as precious on the inside.

I loved having Uncle Foots and Aunt Lorene come up from Florida to spend many holidays with us. She had an extra special surprise for us during one Christmas visit. Exiting the living room to change her outfit, she soon yelled from down the hallway, "Okay, put the music on!" My father did as she'd requested, and Aunt Lorene appeared in a belly dancing outfit! Accustomed to her somewhat quiet demeanor, we were surprised that she'd show her belly, much less belly dance! She not only danced, but Aunt Lorene let it rip, and she was talented. She wore bells on her wrists and ankles, and, oh, did she shimmy!

Lorene was fifty at the time. Clearly, fifty is the age to let it rip! What a role model Aunt Lorene was for doing her own thing and showing us, you are never too old to do what you've always dreamed of doing. Her belly dancing was twofold: a fun hobby to pick up in her fifties and a life-changing health advantage.

Four years after her performance at Christmas, Aunt Lorene and Uncle Foots were enjoying their boat on the ocean at sunset. Just as Uncle Foots was navigating a sharp turn, a huge wave came up and flipped the boat. Both my aunt and uncle were thrown into the water. Uncle Foots had a heart attack and died immediately upon hitting the water. Aunt Lorene knew he had died, yet she held up his body while dog paddling. Incredibly, she continued to tread water for over twelve hours. At sunrise the next morning, two men, who were out for an early morning fishing trip, spotted Aunt Lorene with Uncle Foots and pulled them on their boat.

The event was so traumatizing that Aunt Lorene was hospitalized for days before she could remember her own name, and that's when family was called. The medical team all agreed that belly dancing had saved her life. Her strong stomach muscles and legs had given her the power to tread water while supporting her husband's body.

Be strong, stay active, and move your belly! You never know what you may be called upon to do when you're fifty-plus!

Now, let's not kid ourselves, ladies. This is a turbulent time. That doesn't mean we must drown in despair. We each have a choice. Will you sink, or will you swim?

CHAPTER ONE

A Sticky Situation

"There must be quite a few things a hot bath won't
cure but I don't know many of them."
Sylvia Plath

After school one day, I watched my son intently read a story for an assignment while he waited with me before my doctor's appointment.

"What's so interesting?" I asked. "What are you reading?"
Quickly glancing up, he responded, "'The Great Molasses Flood.'"

I thought he was teasing me. He wasn't, and as we continued to wait together, I began to read over his shoulder. Soon, I was also captivated by the words on the pages.
What comes to mind when you think of molasses? Envisioning Christmas cookies, gingerbread, and cakes, I naturally think of it as the sweet, tasty ingredient in Grandma's goodies. From reading the story, my son and I learned that

molasses has another use. Distilleries turn molasses into rum. Nearly a century ago, a successful Boston distillery was storing large amounts of liquids, including molasses, in huge steel tanks in the business district. They had been operating from that location since 1915, but on January 15, 1919, they gave the residents of Boston a big surprise.

On that day, over two million gallons of molasses were delivered, and, as usual, poured into a huge steel tank at the distillery. All was fine until around noon, when something went terribly wrong. Witnesses recalled hearing a loud popping sound. Suddenly, a fifteen-foot wave of molasses was pouring out into the business district! While the first mental image that comes to mind may resemble a whacky scene from a cartoon episode, the happening was no joke. The sticky wave covered everyone and everything in its way—people, children, and horses—in a terrifying wake of destruction.

I was in a daydream of trying to escape such a scene when the nurse called, "Victoria Teague." Preparing myself for the worst, I almost thought I'd prefer running from molasses. My brain, instead, was racing with several thoughts at once: Why will my food not digest? Why is my workout not working? Why am I getting fat? Why do I not want sex anymore?

I would bombard my doctor—my third doctor so far that year—with the same questions.

My body was changing, and my familiar routines of eating and exercising were no longer working. I felt desperate. I couldn't ignore my suspicion that something was wrong with me—really wrong! I was worried but did not want to say the words aloud. On top of bearing the burden of keeping my fears to myself, I did not feel like myself.

I experienced a brief moment of happiness when my doctor finally entered the exam room and announced, "Healthy, completely healthy!"

Confusion, however, quickly invaded. My emotions were wrapped into one big, complex ball.

"What?" I uttered. "But why am I having all these symptoms?"

"I think you are starting the change in life," he said calmly.

"What change?" I blurted out. "I'm forty-five years old!"

"You are in a stage of life called perimenopause," he said.

"Peri-what? But that's for old women, sometime in the future. Why so early?"

"No," he continued to explain, "you are at the age where women begin to make the change."

"What about my digestive track?" I asked, not a bit confident in his diagnosis.

"Look," he said, speaking as if the answers were really so simple, "I hear this all the time from women your age. Relax, take a hot bath and have a glass of wine. This is the aging process."

Seriously, my third doctor this year and, still, no answers.

"I'll have the nurse come and draw some more blood," he said, placating me, "but I do not think we will find anything."

"Check my thyroid one more time," I insisted. "Please!"

My blood was boiling while waiting for the nurse. I'd spent hours in his office doing a battery of tests, and nothing—nothing showed up. I joined my son, patiently waiting, back in the lobby.

"What happened in Boston?" I asked.

"Oh, Mom, some guy figured out that if they'd use saltwater, the clean-up crew could make greater progress."

Saltwater helped to clean up sticky molasses—amazing!

"Well, maybe that's what I need," I sighed. "Saltwater, if it were only that simple."

My son was too engaged in his story to register what I said.

"Mom, they used saltwater from a fireboat, and the harbor was brown for weeks and weeks."

Where is his teacher going with this assignment? I thought to myself. And what a mess to clean up!

"What caused the molasses blow up?" I was both thinking to myself and asking my son.
"They thought it was the unusually warm weather for January that year," he eagerly shared. "But it turned out that the construction of the steel tanks and low maintenance caused the metal pins of the containers to bust, and the walls were no longer supported!"

I could hear the excitement in his voice before his tone grew more serious.

"Twenty-one adults, two children, and two horses died. Another one hundred fifty were injured, all due to a lack of proper maintenance."

As we checked out and left the doctor's office, that molasses story stuck in my head. Later, I called my friend Adrienne who was a few years older than I. Free to release my pent-up frustration, I spouted off about how ignorant all my doctors had been.

"What kind of specialist do you have to find?" I asked. "I need answers!"

Like a good friend, she heard the exasperation in my voice and let me vent. When I was ready to listen, she assured me, saying,

"There, there, darlin', it's all gonna work out!"

My real-deal, Southern (from Charleston, South Carolina) girlfriend left me with a little beacon of hope.

Typically a healthy lady who rarely went to the doctor, Adrienne had endured a four-year period of being diagnosed with irritable bowel syndrome (IBS), heart palpitations, dizzy spells, insomnia, low-functioning thyroid, depression and no sex drive. How does a healthy person end up with so many problems in four years? That's enough to make a person crazy! How many doctors can you go to? Thankfully for Adrienne, someone suggested that she have her hormones checked and found all symptoms were linked to menopause. Prescribed a few herbal remedies and a low dose of hormone replacement therapy (HRT), Adrienne had her good health back within a month or so.

I was so happy for my dear friend and of course, thought my story would mimic hers. With Adrienne guiding me, I began my journey into the world of alternative medicine through a natural clinic near us. I'd simply been going to the wrong sources, I thought, and would now be restored to my former self. Little did I know, it would not turn out quite so simply for me.

Fast forward five years. I was fifty years old and still on a hellacious ride after visiting every natural specialist in town and throwing thousands of dollars down the toilet. Despite every agonizing symptom, I had not yet reached menopause. No, I was in perimenopause. Would it ever end? Day after day, alone with my thoughts during the quiet hours of the afternoon before my husband and children returned home, I'd feel like screaming. Would I ever get off this nightmarish rollercoaster?

I'm not sure what caused my transformation. Whether from the stomach/digestive disorder, the weight gain, the disrupted workouts or the fatigue, somewhere along the line, I turned in my Superwoman cape and started behaving like a victim. Every little thing bothered me—greatly. My emotions led me from sobbing to raging and back to sobbing. I would tell my husband this wasn't me. My husband would tell me to find another specialist. He simply did not know what else to do or say.

On one day, going about my business, I suddenly experienced heart palpitations. Not only did my heart feel strange, but a tremendous darkness also came with it. Am I having a heart attack? I wasn't sure. Do I call someone? I felt dizzy and broke into a sweat. I got on Google (oh, do that if you want to become really scared!) and was convinced I was having a heart attack. I called my husband, who left work to take me to the emergency room.

I remember being whizzed to the back quickly and hooked up to several different machines. Next, they tossed a host of questions at me so rapidly my head was spinning. About five minutes into the emergency room frenzy of activity, everyone calmed down. By the reactions of the staff, I could tell my case was not an emergency. Much later, the doctor reviewed several tests and concluded that I had inflammation in my chest muscles.

The doctor asked, "Have you been lifting any heavy weights lately?"

We all burst out laughing. "Do I look like I've been lifting weights?" I asked. "I'm fifty years old and twenty-five pounds overweight."

"Have you been doing strenuous yard work?"

"No," I said with a chuckle.

"You have inflammation in your chest muscles," he concluded without any explanation. "Do not do any heavy lifting or anything unusual and take this for a week."

He prescribed a strong version of ibuprofen. Despite having no answers, three hours later, my husband and I were on our way home, delighted to know my heart was fine.

After the ordeal, a hot bath was calling my name. Soaking in the tub and listening to my meditation music, I let my tears flow freely.

"Dear God, will this season ever pass?" I cried out.

When I heard Jeff, my husband, coming into the bedroom, I tried to quiet my sobs. The thoughts continued. My daughter is graduating in six weeks from high school. I'm overwhelmed with symptoms, and I still have no answers. Jeff poked his head into the bathroom.

"Are you okay?" he asked.

"No!" I shouted, releasing sobs. "I've had . . . *sob* . . . a huge . . . *sob* . . . molasses spill . . . *sob, sob, sob* . . . and I don't . . . *sob, sob* . . . have any . . . *sob* . . . saltwater!"

"I don't have a clue what you are talking about," he replied as calmly as humanly possible, "but let's think about some counseling tomorrow. Okay, hon?"

"Oh, thanks, honey!" I shot back. "Now you want me to see a shrink! Oh, and by the way, I'm a psych major, if you don't mind!"

On a positive note, I still had a little spunk in me!

Does any of this sound familiar to you? Many of us experience a huge host of symptoms as we go through the period of our life called perimenopause, leading into meno-pause. No matter our symptoms, most of us are caught off guard.

No one forewarned me. No one talked about it or tried to prepare me for what was coming. Nevertheless, as I got still and prayed that night in my tub, I had a revelation: God moves in mysterious ways. A flash of energy stirred in my spirit and that crazy molasses flood story lingered in my brain. Suddenly, I had a single thought: Who says you don't have saltwater? It was coming from somewhere deep within. My soul knew that I had saltwater. Yes, indeed, God moves in mysterious ways.

As I prayed, it occurred to me that the molasses came in a gigantic wave. Initially, it made a big mess. That mess resulted because of a lack of maintenance. The cleanup then progressed slowly until someone suggested a solution: saltwater.

"I've cracked the code! I've cracked the code!" I shouted from the bath.

My husband, calling his reply to me from downstairs, said, "Okay honey, whatever you say! I'm glad you cracked the code."

I slid down into my hot bubble bath, and a deep comfort came over me. It was unexplainable, supernatural. Knowing there was hope, I felt a profound shift within my spirit.

Finding Your Saltwater

Many women around the age of forty-five experience a gigantic mess of symptoms that have poured into our bodies. Before that happens, we are proud of our lives. We acknowledge that we've accomplished so much.

Can you stop right now and applaud yourself?

While possibly experiencing the joys of raising your family, and perhaps excelling in the marketplace or a chosen profession, you could easily see and feel how God was blessing you in those seasons. You put all your systems in place, and they worked. Then, out of nowhere, the pins popped, and you were left with a big mess!

I know. You do not feel like you have the energy to deal with it, but you do. You have the strength—a deep, inner strength. You will see! I'm confident that you will.

Looking back, I now see where God blessed me richly, but my past health was not perfect. I was not eating a nutritious, balanced diet. Thin, I appeared in good shape, but I pushed myself relentlessly. I worked out for hours in the gym to keep up my "lean, mean machine," and my approach worked throughout my thirties and into my early forties. I took great pride in my workouts. I took great pride in my fast-paced lifestyle, which included my children's schedules. It all worked as I raised two beautiful kids and ran a charity, but at the age of forty-five, my body crashed.

I could no longer keep up with the long cardio workouts and heavy weight programs. I became anemic as my cycles changed, which is why I almost passed out while lifting weights at the gym one day. That's when I realized it was time to get into the doctor's office, thereby launching my long search from doctor to doctor and clinic to clinic. I ended up with a huge box of supplements, protein drinks, magnesium, natural progesterone, and a wide range of diets. Nothing really worked, however. I would feel better briefly, only to have the same problems return or an entirely different set of symptoms flare up. All the while, I was burning through money, desperate to figure this out. The hit on my pocketbook made everything more stressful.

Now—finally—I have found my saltwater.

Can you imagine being the first clean-up crew to come in after that gigantic wave of molasses hit the streets of Boston? Where would you begin? This menopausal journey feels much like that molasses wave as your body fluctuates with hormonal changes. You may be asking, which symptom do I treat? It's all so confusing.

How are we going to clean up this gigantic mess?

As for Boston, the cleanup in the immediate area took weeks and more than three hundred hardworking folks to make it happen. The surrounding area took a great deal longer. Imagine the crew and commuters attempting to get through it as they tracked the goo with each step. Trains, subways, even telephone booths were left with a sticky coating. Can you imagine everything you touched being sticky for months? Apparently, on hot summer days in the decades following the tragedy, people could smell a hint of molasses.

I want you to master this season and do it well. My goal is for you to succeed and never, ever think about hanging up your Superwoman's cape! You are still a super woman, oh yeah! A super woman with wisdom.

I know it's been hell, my friend, so let's find heaven. I have traversed this passage and I have found the saltwater! I have cracked the menopausal code and I'm here to share my secrets! Let's get started with this sticky mess, shall we?

CHAPTER TWO

Brain Fog City

"Life is like a jigsaw puzzle, you have to see the
whole picture, then put it together piece by piece."
Terry McMillan

The party was everything we had hoped for: great turnout, perfect location, beautiful weather. It was just the right temperature for a May evening in the South. What a celebration for my daughter's sweet sixteenth birthday!

After we loaded up our cars and said our final goodbyes, every car exited the country club until only two of us were left. The other person was my friend who had cohosted the celebration that our two daughters, long-time friends, had shared. I was in my vehicle and my friend was in hers. Separated from everyone else, we had both pulled behind the clubhouse, which was right next to the golf course, for final loading of the decor and leftover cake. Excited to share the news of the night with another close girlfriend, I immediately jumped on my phone as I drove off.

In the midst of gabbing, I didn't realize I'd veered onto a side road. Vaguely, I remembered following the headlights from my friend's car as she'd left, but I suddenly had no idea where I was. It was midnight, pitch black, and I couldn't see a thing. I promptly ended the phone conversation to concentrate on where I was going. Suddenly, a loud *scre-e-e-e-e-ch* pierced the darkness. I slammed on my brakes and then tried to open my car door. I couldn't. A low, stone wall prevented me from escaping!

Deep breath, Victoria. Deep breath. Don't panic!

It was very, very dark—frighteningly dark.

Okay, do not panic, I tried to convince myself. Frustrated and nervous all at once, I called the first person who would certainly come to my rescue: my husband. And his phone was off! Next, I called my son. No answer! I called my daughter.

She answered, and I shouted, "I'm in a very bad spot!"

"Where are you?" She asked. "We're all pulling up the driveway, home."

"Don't ask," I said. "I might need you guys to come back to the clubhouse."

Before I could say another word, car lights appeared from below. They were headed towards me.

Terrified, I blurted, "Hannah, I'm hanging up and calling 9-1-1. I'll call you back."

Yikes! I imagined all the people wondering whatever happened to Victoria Teague and how on earth did her car end up in that strange spot! Seconds later, a van pulled up in front of me, shining its lights on my car. Sheer terror struck before I heard the familiar voice of my friend and party cohost.

"Hey, did you make the wrong turn, too?" she asked. Relief poured over me, and then we both chuckled.

"What did we do?" I called to her.

She shouted over her car engine, "I don't know, but you are getting ready to scrape your car up really bad."

"What?" I had no idea what she meant.

"You are stuck on a stone-laden bridge on the golf course! These bridges are sized for golf carts."

By simply following her, instead of paying attention, I'd ended up on the narrow golf cart route that circled the course.

"Aw-w-w!" I moaned, thinking how I dreaded sharing this news with Jeff. "How do we get out?"

She gave me the bad news.

"There's no way out down here. You have to scrape your car by coming on through. Come down the hill, circle around, and come back over the bridge you are on for a second time. Oh, and be careful. There's a huge drop-off down here. I almost went over the cliff!"

I came on through the bridge: *scrape . . . screech . . . screech . . . screech*. Oh, man, Jeff is going to kill me! That was all I could think about. After the first tight squeeze, scraping up the car pretty badly, I swung around to make the circle. I followed my friend for yet another tight squeeze to go back across the tiny little stone bridge made for golf carts. Talk about getting your adrenaline up! My only consolation: at least two of us did it!

And, of course, my family, plus all the friends of my children who were spending the night, were waiting on the driveway when I pulled up to my home. They could not wait to see this one! Brain, where did you go? We had a good laugh, and so did many others, as our story became the talk among our circle of friends and though the kids' school. Thankfully, the car was able to be buffed out on both sides, so no harm done. My ego was bruised a little, but you know what we women are—resilient!

We women are resilient in our own right.

Webster's Dictionary defines resilient as *"able to become strong, healthy, or successful again after something bad happens"* and *"to return to an original shape after being pulled, stretched, pressed, bent, etc."*

What a description of menopause!

You're probably aware of perimenopause and menopause, and you may be all too familiar with many of the symptoms, including brain fog and the physical signs that accompany this life-changing time! Even so, a brief review of a few main ideas can reinforce what you may have already experienced and prepare you for what you may expect. Take a deep breath and relax.

To uncover the seven secrets that will help you make this passage, it's good to review the process in steps.

View the Big Picture

The first step is to take a step back to view the big picture as an observer. You're gathering information. What are your symptoms? What do your symptoms point out to you? Your body is highly intelligent. It will tell you what it needs as you sit back and listen. Getting a feel for what is going on with the right information will enhance your understanding. In fact, your body will give you a map to find your way out of this menopause mayhem.

Let's start with the basics of what is happening and how your hormones play a role.

According to Webster's Dictionary, menopause is, *"the definitive end of a woman's menstrual cycle,"* which comes from the French word *ménopause,* which from the Latin *menopausis.* Interestingly, menopause incorporates the word *pause,* suggesting that menstruation may resume, when it does not.

The average age for women to reach their last period is about fifty-two, but some women go through it as early as forty and some as late as fifty-eight, give or take a few years. I have heard an occasional nightmare story, including that of my grandmother, who had her period until age seventy. She gave birth to twelve children, and the doctor believed that the high number of births led to her unusually late menopausal season. While an extreme example, she died a healthy lady, which should not be a surprise. The longer the ovaries function, the longer organs like the heart benefit from the production of estrogen. My grandmother simply went to sleep at ninety-three and never woke up—a peaceful, quiet passing for an elegant woman.

Menopause is *not* a medical crisis even though some might refer to it as a mid-life crisis. Truly, it's just a natural part of life. The entire process of saying goodbye to your cycle can last from six to thirteen years, so you must get used to the process as a stage in life! Menopause is the time in a woman's life when menstrual periods permanently stop; it is also called the "change of life." Menopause is defined as the time when there have been no menstrual periods for twelve consecutive months and no other biological or physiological cause can be identified.

Now, if like most, you probably remember the day you got your period. No doubt, it was a big ordeal. However, tracking your last period is a bit more complicated. Unless you've had a hysterectomy, you most likely don't know for sure when the last one was, but you can guess. Although a guessing game, eventually you'll figure it out. After arriving into menopause, making it a year without a period, hormones do tend to level back out and you'll figure out your new normal. There's much you can do in perimenopause that I'm so excited to share with you!

Menopausal symptoms are quite a bothersome ordeal for some, but other women seem to sail through the menopausal transition with flying colors. They call it "much ado about nothing!" and we hate those ladies, don't we! *Smile*. For most women, perimenopause is the season referred as ***hormonal hell.***

In either case, nothing lasts forever. Symptoms are at their height during perimenopause, but then taper off and usually disappear altogether within a year or so after the last period.

A Range of Symptoms

From researching information presented by Dr. Christiane Northrup, M.D., as well as doctors Edward A. Taub, M.D., F.A.A.P. and Ferid Murad, M.D., PhD., I offer a rundown of the most common symptoms reported during "the change," although please keep in mind that certainly not all women experience all of them.

Brain Fog is a temporary effect of the hormonal changes of perimenopause. Symptoms include difficulty concentrating and minor forgetfulness. The situation is similar to the mental fuzziness many women experience after giving birth; scattered thinking is designed to turn your attention inward so that you can focus on yourself for a change. After years of multitasking, possibly juggling children and careers, it's time to stop and pay attention to yourself.

Hot flashes are the most common symptom of perimenopause, experienced to some degree by up to eighty-five percent of women. Hot flashes reach their height near the end of perimenopause. Many women also have night sweats that are severe enough to wake them regularly, disrupting their sleep. Night sweats tend to occur between 3:00 and 4:00 a.m. for most women, although those who stay up extra late at night or who work night shifts may experience a different pattern. Hot flashes and night sweats are more severe in women who are under emotional stress, as well as in women who eat a diet high in simple sugars and refined carbohydrates found in baked goods, candy, white bread, white potatoes, white pasta, wine, liquor, and beer. They are also far more common in women who've had hysterectomies—with or without ovary removal.

Mood swings, such as irritability and depression, are also typical hallmarks of perimenopause. They are especially troublesome for women who previously experienced mood swings before their periods.

Irregular periods are the first sign that the menopausal transition has begun, which typically happens anywhere from two to eight years before a woman's last menstrual period. In fact, women who have previously been as regular as clockwork may go for several months without a period. Even though the irregular periods are a signal that you aren't ovulating every month, that doesn't mean you aren't ovulating at all. Lighter and heavier flow during periods are both common.

Breast tenderness can occur more frequently in women who previously experienced premenstrual tenderness. Breast tenderness is often a sign of iodine deficiency, too.

Insomnia, with or without night sweats, can occur at this time.

Heart palpitations during the menopausal transition are experienced by women with higher levels of stress hormones caused by, among other things, greater levels of fear and anxiety. Often, the sensations arise from past trauma that you now have the strength to resolve once and for all. Heart palpitations can also be a sign of thyroid imbalance. Chest pain (angina), another possible symptom, is related both to stress hormones and lack of progesterone.

Migraines may occur more often in perimenopause, usually (but not always) in women who previously experienced migraines before their period. They are often triggered by falling progesterone levels.

Hypothyroidism, which often has no overt symptoms and can be diagnosed only with proper testing, occurs in up to one quarter of women at this time. In many women, the condition is caused by iodine deficiency. Be sure to have a doctor monitor your thyroid hormone levels.

Benign uterine fibroids, or non-cancerous tumors made up of muscle and connective tissue, develop in about forty percent of women.

Changes in sex drive are also common. Contrary to popular belief, the hormone changes during menopause don't lower sex drive in healthy women. For some women, however, a drop in testosterone, whether from drugs, surgery, or adrenal exhaustion, can reduce sexual desire. Changes in estrogen levels also reduce sex drive in some, in addition to causing vaginal dryness and irritation that make intercourse painful. This can be easily alleviated with lubricants or topical estrogen creams available by prescription. For women who've reached the one-year mark without a period, however, the freedom from the worry of unwanted pregnancy can be one factor in heightening sex drive.

Bone loss can be a problem, especially for women who don't eat a nutritious diet and fail to exercise. Bone loss is also a sign of vitamin D deficiency. All women should have their vitamin D levels checked.

Brain chemistry also changes in midlife, affecting the way women think and process information. For example, midlife women often find that they not only have stronger feelings about injustice and unfairness, but they're also more willing to speak up about these feelings. Because the temporal lobes in the brain are more often engaged, intuition is enhanced. Interestingly, unlike most of the symptoms in the previous list, the shifts in brain chemistry are permanent—a sign that women really do get wiser as life progresses. Numerous studies substantiate this theory. The book *Switch on Your Brain* by Dr. Caroline Leaf is a great source for explaining the changes in brain chemistry.

You may also find that you have a much stronger creative

drive since your energy isn't being used to have periods and create babies. Instead, it gets rerouted into powerful urges to create. You may feel compelled to pick up a musical instrument, write, sing, paint, birth a thriving new business, or exercise. How about belly dancing! Long-buried dreams and feelings resurface with a renewed passion at this time. It's as if your soul is saying, hey, what about me? When is it my turn?

If you don't act on your innermost dreams and desires now and, instead, hold them in, then you're apt to have a much harder time with menopausal symptoms. But that's not all: According to Dr. Northrup in her book *The Wisdom of Menopause*, you may be setting yourself up for health problems. The bottom line is that women are designed to be more in touch with what really matters after menopause. Your body, therefore, acts as an incredibly accurate barometer that indicates how closely you're living your life in line with your true heart's desires. Often, this is a calling that was put on the back burner as your children or career became front and center. It's now time for you to go deep within and look forward to birthing a new season.

Jacquelyn's Story

I had met Jacquelyn while working on a project with my foundation. It was truly a divine connection, as neither of us knew the season that would blow in on us and subsequent reasons we were sent to one another.

When I looked at Jacquelyn's life, my head would spin. She juggled so many responsibilities! I had observed her working on a project with my foundation, and she ran the show beautifully. I also saw firsthand how adeptly she performed her role as an advertising executive. Helping my daughter Hannah with a class project, Jacquelyn had graciously allowed the two of us to spend an afternoon sitting in on several meetings at her marketing agency. I was amazed as Jacquelyn flowed effortlessly from one meeting to the next, all the while giving orders, delegating plans, and discussing new marketing strategies. In addition, she was raising three beautiful teens, a daughter and two boys, each only two years apart in age.

I asked her how she did it. Head of a marketing firm, mother of three teenagers, and wife of a husband with a corporate career as well, Jacquelyn was my cool friend from California.

When she invited me to lunch at her home, I imagined that the place would be immaculate, and it was. Everything was in order and flawlessly decorated with gorgeous plants and vibrant, rich colors. As I sunk onto the coach while waiting for Jacqulyn to return with tea, I had time to admire a heavenly painting on the wall. So light and airy with grey and teal highlights, it reminded me of the best sunny day at the beach.

Absorbing my surroundings, I found myself melting into the cozy couch. It all was so lovely! Oh, to live like that! It seemed that my friend had the perfect life.

When Jacquelyn returned and poured our tea, I made a point of sitting up and taking special care with my cup. Despite being preoccupied with not making a mess, I noted that my friend was not her perky, energetic self. As soon as I said so, Jacquelyn let her bottled-up concerns spill out.

"I'm not feeling well. I don't have the normal energy levels that I've had all these years. I can't figure out what is going on. I'm exhausted all the time."

Quickly, I put on my counselor's hat.

"Let's take a deeper look at the entire picture," I said.

I instinctively began to think that she might be lugging around some emotional baggage. If left unchecked, if she were not tending to her heart and soul, it would be sapping her energy.

"You do so much, Jacquelyn," I said. "Can we slow down and look a little deeper at what's going on under the hood?"

A gentle smile from me was all the encouragement my distraught friend required.

Our lunch turned into a three-hour counseling session. Jacquelyn communicated that she was over-committed and undernourished. A high-powered executive running the show, she was not listening to the vital cues her body was trying to share with her.

"Jacquelyn," I said, "you've got to slow down and regroup so you can continue to move forward. Your body is changing and shifting, and you must make the change with it. Otherwise," I continued, "you will see your body as an enemy. Your body wants to work with you during this season, but it's telling you it's exhausted."

I gestured towards all the eye-catching elements around the room.

"Look at all this beauty around you," I said. "Are you enjoying it?"

I knew her answer, no.

"You are flying through your life so fast, you are missing vital cues. I don't want you to end up sick."

As she shook her head in agreement with me, she still had a look of desperation in her eyes. Her heart was saying, yes,

Victoria, I agree with you, but her head was fighting the idea of how will I hang onto this life I've built if I slow down. A look of fear radiated in her eyes.

"With some planning and delegating, you can figure this out," I assured her.

I felt great concern for Jacquelyn as we ended our lunch and said our goodbyes. The few panicked phone calls I received from her later were not a surprise. Throughout, I tried my best to comfort and encourage her to get off the crazy treadmill of frenzied activity that she described to me. She needed to make some key choices about her priorities, but Jacquelyn did not change anything.

The fallout in her life started with a lack of energy. Jacquelyn was the sharp, go-to person for everyone: family, work, community, and friends. If someone needed a contact, she could pull the person's name and number right off the top of her head. With her knack for numbers, she could do math in her head and tell you if the deal was going to work. She instinctively knew if something would be profitable.

As perimenopause ripped its way into Jacquelyn's life, however, she started making mistakes. For the first time, simple dates got jumbled in her mind. She could not snap out of a perpetual fog. At the same time, she was putting on weight, which her husband mentioned. He's what I'd classify as a Type-A personality. Since Jacquelyn was a strong, independent type herself, his comments about her weight hit a wrong nerve and infuriated her. The constant nagging about getting her weight down became too much. She also did not have her previously high-energy levels to maintain her long workouts. Things that she normally could have brushed off really agitated her.

Finally, the day came when she could no longer take her husband's criticism, and her business partner stepped in as

her white knight. An older man, he'd suffered his own difficult period when his wife had passed away a few years before.
During Jacquelyn's tough time, he had been her deeply com-
mitted ally, always providing a shoulder on which to cry. He
was compassionate and, being older, understood the changes
Jacquelyn was experiencing. His caring ear and comforting
advice were the opposite of her husband's impatience, lack of
insight, and criticism. Besides, as a younger woman, despite
gaining a few extra pounds, she remained attractive to the
older man. All along, her emotional state grew more and more
erratic with mood swings that affected other aspects of her
normally responsible and dependable behavior.

She began leaning on him more heavily, and as her marriage
continued to deteriorate, her relationship at the office heated
up. One night, after work, he invited her to dinner. After
several glasses of wine, the invitation to his home for dessert
was enticing. A glass of brandy and a neck rub naturally led to
the next thing, and they found themselves in bed together. It
felt so right, but it was so wrong. By the next morning, they
had each recognized the big mistake, and this led to further
complications at work.

His comforting ear at the office became distant and aloof.
The business suffered as her brain fog increased. All along,
her emotional state grew more and more erratic, and her
outbursts became the common theme around the office. The
final straw was her blowing up on their number one client.
Losing the account removed one-third of the company's reve-
nues. Likewise, her business partner was looking for a way to
buy her out. The board of directors wanted Jacquelyn out as
well. The pressure was immense. People started avoiding her.

While Jacquelyn's business was falling apart, her husband
of twenty-five years was asking for a divorce. I'll never forget
the day she called to tell me.

As Jacquelyn sobbed on the phone with me, she communicated that she physically felt horrible. Her energy had

bottomed out. Before she had finally been bought out for much less than the business had originally been worth, she was exhausted and leaving work early. Since selling, she was spending her days sleeping.

The last thing to go was her digestive track. She reacted violently to everything she put in her mouth. Her hypersensitive reactions were not only strange and varied, but also inconsistent. She could eat blueberries on one day and be fine; the next time, Jacquelyn would respond as if allergic to them.

Physically and emotionally drained, she could no longer hold a job. Instead, she was spending money as she went from doctor to doctor, and health clinic to health clinic, yet getting no answers. Making it more unbearable, her children blamed her as word got out that she had an affair. Her life caved in, creating a dark place for Jacquelyn.

The sharp, powerful woman—the one who had birthed a business, enriched her community, and perfectly filled the roles of super mom and trophy wife—burned and crashed hard. On top of everything, news about her husband's leaving was spreading throughout the community; the gossip grapevine was buzzing.

What pitfalls could Jacquelyn have avoided on her way to hormonal hell?

When I met Jacquelyn, in her late thirties at the time, I viewed her life like a beautiful bouquet of flowers. I wasn't seeing everything. If it had been so wonderful, even the most spectacular flowers die. Withering flowers don't have to end up in the trash; they can be made into a lovely dried arrangement, but they are never truly the same.

You may prefer to view your life as a garden, and gardens must be tended. Think about having the right soil and planting conditions. Watering and appropriate sunlight also go hand in hand. Don't forget those pesky weeds. You must weed out what no longer works. To determine which people and things are weeds, consider what drains your life of vibrancy. Doing what's right for your garden requires that you adjust for each season.

Balancing Life's Spiritual, Mental, Physical, and Social Components

To counsel Jacquelyn, I faced a big molasses spill. Where would we start? Author Stephen Covey's *The 7 Habits of Highly Successful People* offers a model for keeping life in balance. My version stipulates that you must tend to four areas of life: Spiritual, Mental, Physical, and Social. Look at each one as a drawer that you must open, inspect, clear out, rearrange, and restock daily to stay in balance.

1) Spiritual: checking in with your spiritual source each day
2) Mental: exercising your mind at work or school
3) Physical: moving your body
4) Social: staying connected to a supportive Tribe; not isolating

By inspecting each aspect of life each day, you'll notice which parts of your life are in order and balanced, and which need the most work. Take time to bring each area into alignment for your highest good. Make the effort to become your best for you and for everyone else in your life.

Jacquelyn's story isn't over. There's more to come.

Tend to the garden of your life. While you're at it, give yourself permission to chuckle at your brain fog stories. I'm still laughing at mine and thankful that my car is in one piece!

Saltwater Tip: Choice and personal responsibility are keys to unlocking a Joyous Menopause. Readjusting your life in each season is essential. Balancing your Spiritual, Mental, Physical, and Social aspects of life delivers big rewards.

CHAPTER THREE

French Fry or Die!
Give Me Those Fries!

"When diet is wrong, medicine is of no use. When
diet is correct, medicine is of no need."
Ancient Ayurvedic Proverb

She must have been famished! The woman rushed into
McDonald's and eagerly pushed her way up through the
line. "I'll have a large order of fries!" she snapped at the young
lady behind the counter. McDonald's was packed; it was the
lunch rush on a holiday. Tons of children were buzzing around
the playground area while moms, chatting with one another,
watched from nearby booths.

"Ma'am, it will be a few minutes on your fries," the young
lady working the counter replied because the fry bin was
empty. "Can you step to the side?"

The woman, who looked to be in her early fifties, stepped
aside. More customers came up and ordered. French fries were
soon ready, but they went out to all the other customers. The

31

neglected woman began to pace. Finally, after a ten-minute wait of watching many others walking off with their French fry orders, she charged the counter. As she climbed over, one of her high heels flew off and almost hit a nearby child. Undeterred, she grabbed a perfectly cooked French fry from the staging area.

"What does this look like!" she screamed, shaking it at the young lady who had taken her order. "What is this?" she demanded.

A F-French fry?" the young worker stammered.
"And what do I look like?" the customer asked.
"A . . . customer?" the employee answered.

At this point the manager, appeared from the back of the kitchen and approached the crime scene. The busy restaurant grew quiet, and all eyes were on the main characters.

"Okay, lady," the manager said, "we will get you some free fries," as he ushered her back to the other side of the counter.

He picked up her high heel pump, and as he handed it to her, she grabbed it and broke off the already loose heel. Leaving the manager with his mouth gaping open, the woman then burst into tears and ran out of the McDonald's, throwing the heel to the ground.

My friends and I chuckled, and then promptly told our kids never to behave like that in a restaurant. I felt a tad sorry for a grown woman who'd had a tantrum over French fries, but I honestly couldn't relate to her problem. What was her deal? A major carb carving, evidently, and a bruised ego, or was it something much deeper? Had she been overlooked her entire life? I was guessing that her tantrum wasn't only about fries.

Cravings vs. Nutritious Consumption

Today, I could write a book, much less a chapter, about cravings versus nutritious consumption during this perimenopausal/

menopausal season. Food is such an important piece of the puzzle now, as in every season. You should strive to eat as many nutritious options as possible for your health. No more of the yo-yo dieting that so many of us have been prone to do!

The goal is to help you figure out a lifestyle plan that works for the long haul. I personally went through a long, frustrating season of watching my weight soar higher and higher. I could not crack the code on my eating during perimenopause. The combination of unexplained weight gain and feeling helpless to get it off is one of the reasons why many women become depressed during this season. Yes, hormonal imbalances come into play, and your food choices affect how you feel and your overall wellbeing.

As an old Irish proverb says, "Laughter is brightest where food is best."

Again, it took me ten years of frustration, tears, giving up, and then giving the effort another shot to crack this complex code. To start, you must understand how your body flourishes in menopause. At that point, you'll have insights to pick up some tips and options to become the best you.

A Paleo Diet

Towards the end of perimenopause, I adopted a Paleo diet and have not looked back. Living a Paleo lifestyle means eating foods that your body recognizes as food. The philosophy contends that food is best when it's as close to its natural state as possible. That means going back in time to the days of the hunter-gatherer—yes, caveman days! What would they eat? I need only to go back to my grandmothers' generation. They cooked all their food from scratch and often pulled the vegetables right out of their backyard gardens. Both of mine lived into their nineties.

Would Grandmother have eaten this? That's a great question to ask yourself, although a Paleo diet has some essential components:

33

- Grass-fed meats, wild-caught fish and seafood

- Healthy, natural fats like coconut oil, avocado, grass-fed butters, and olive oil

- A wide variety of organic vegetables

- Organic fruits

- Pasture-fed eggs and dairy
  Note: It's best to avoid dairy if you have an autoimmune disease or are trying to lose weight.

- Nuts and seeds in moderation

- Natural sweeteners, such as raw, organic honey, pure organic maple syrup or stevia
  Note: It's best to avoid sweeteners and/or use only a little honey or syrup if you're aiming to lose weight.

Paleo plans exclude grains, legumes, soy, vegetable oils, refined sugars, artificial colors and sweeteners, and highly processed foods.

What I love about Paleo is that it's not only a diet, but a lifestyle. The practice is about simplifying your life to make time for food and the things you love the most, whether family, hobbies, work, or exercise. A healthy lifestyle involves many factors, not only food. If you start with food, however, you'll be willing and able to address the other areas of your life that are making you unhealthy and unhappy.

I hope that makes sense to you. After I cracked the food code, the rest fell into place.

How to Make Paleo the Simple Option

Let's face it: The world is stressful and downright hectic because of the schedules we choose. That's why the first step is to simplify. Whether reducing work hours or decluttering your home, choose to push back the layers that do not matter. Simplifying your life can feel like a huge weight coming off. It's a must in this season!

How does cleaning up your diet relate to simplifying, especially if you are no longer opening cans and boxes to make those quick-and-easy recipes?

To be honest, I'm a terrible cook, and my husband and kids joke about it often. That's probably because I've been somewhat of a lazy cook. I've spent years relying on quick meals, often grabbing them to eat on the go because of our family members' schedules. Even now that my kids are older, I'm still not the person who's going to spend hours on end in the kitchen.

Does this register for you? If so, a little planning keeps Paleo simple.

Make a weekly or monthly menu. By planning and jotting down your menu for the week or even the month, you'll know what to buy and what to take out of the freezer. You'll avoid the most popular questions starting at 5:00 p.m.: *What's for dinner, Mom? Honey, what do we have to eat tonight?* Shopping ahead based on your menus also fights the temptations of driving to the fast-food window, picking up Chinese takeout, or grabbing a bag of chips. The urge to eat anything skyrockets before the dinner hour. Planning a menu keeps you out of the danger zone of snacking or grabbing wrong choices before dinner.

Buy the food. The concept sounds simple enough, but when your schedule is busy, you must slow down to think about your menu and make a grocery list for the ingredients. Scheduling time for the planning and the shopping helps you avoid going back and forth to the store throughout the week. That is a timesaver. You may also be surprised that planning your weekly menu takes less than an hour. If your local store allows you to order your food ahead of time online, then all you have to do is go there to pick up the items, bagged and ready. How great is that? Likewise, if you have delivery options, you may calculate that the time you save is worth any additional cost.

Take time to prep. By prepping ingredients in advance, you'll save time. How much extra time does it take to chop two onions instead of one? Twenty seconds? Keep your freezer stocked with such ingredients to use them quickly at a later time. Also, double up on batches of sauce or meat. Freeze and pull out what you need when needed. Having the right foods on hand can encourage you to stick with nutritious meals. How hard is it to go your freezer? If time had been your number one excuse for avoiding a Paleo plan, then you now have three simple tips that will end up saving time and making you feel better and more satisfied.

I spent ten years in perimenopause with horrible digestive tract issues. Multiple doctors could never quite figure out the problem. They settled for the IBS (irritable bowel syndrome) family. I tried diet after diet to no accord; the issues of extreme bloating and swelling and weight gain were still there. No amount of exercise would budge the weight. I was so frustrated yet refused to give up. In searching, I discovered fasting.

Saltwater Tip: Intermittent fasting promotes healing.

Why Fast?

With all the dieting advice out there, you may be thinking that the easiest approach is simply not to eat. Fasting for your health, however, is not the same as starving yourself. Also, fasting is not a diet, although the concept of abstaining from food and drink for a specific period has been around for thousands of years. Spiritual fasting is also a part of many religions.

When fasting for your health, instead of consuming three square meals or several small meals throughout the day, you would have a few hours of a day or certain days of the week when you'd eat. During that time, you would eat whatever you wanted. Of course, "whatever you want" is within reason.

If you're eating processed foods and potato chips, you probably won't reap the benefits of fasting. In that case, I'd encourage you to examine your diet before trying a fast. If you'll mostly consume a diet of whole food, rich in fruits, veggies, lean proteins, healthy fats, and raw dairy, then you'll see the beneficial changes from fasting. In fact, the occasional splurges on chocolate or cheese won't have as big of an impact as they might if you were on a calorie-restrictive diet.

Different Types of Fasting

The question of how to fast is wide open. The beauty of fasting is that there isn't one right way to do it. You'll also find several popular types of fasting from which to choose. Experts like Dr. Josh Axe, DNM, DC, CNS offer a variety of fasting options that you can find online.

Intermittent fasting entails refraining from solid foods during certain periods of time according to a specific schedule. Time-restricted fasting, a form of intermittent fasting, stipulates that you would not eat anything during longer periods, usually twelve to sixteen hours in the day. A 16:8 fast, for instance, would have you fast for sixteen consecutive hours of the day. If you implemented alternate-day fasting, you would severely restrict your diet every other day. A 5:2 diet stipulates eating normally for five days and greatly restricting calories on the other two days. A warrior diet would restrict your foods to fruits and vegetables during the day with one well-balanced meal at night.

Finally, the Daniel Fast—a spiritual fast based on Daniel's experiences from the Bible's Book of Daniel—is a partial fast that allows vegetables, fruits and other healthy whole foods, but no meat, dairy, or grains unless they're sprouted ancient grains. Also, drinks like coffee, alcohol and juice are avoided.

Most people follow this fast for twenty-one days to experience a spiritual breakthrough, reflect on their relationship with God, or feel closer to what Daniel would have experienced in his time.

My Breakdown-to-Breakthrough Moment

Shortly after beginning my paleo nutrition plan, I began a twenty-one-day Daniel Fast with a group. I chose only organic options and limited my fruit. Be careful with fruit, which has sugar—deadly to the body in this season!

During our spiritual Daniel Fast, my friends and I stayed in prayer and meditation more than usual, meaning we focused our thoughts on God as much as possible. It was day seventeen of the fast when I experienced an unforgettable moment. About to enter our local Sprouts for groceries, I had the strangest pulling and popping sensation in my lower throat area on the left side, the exact location of my thyroid.

After the sensation left, I had a burst of energy! I believe my thyroid was healed at that very moment. In other words, that slugged-out, exhausted feeling, which I'd endured for ten years, lifted permanently and never came back!

From fasting, you may question how the healing occurred. Could it have been the nutrient-rich juices that were feeding the cells, while allowing my body the opportunity to detoxify? Or was it a direct act of God? I think the answer is simple. Whether from the miracle of fasting or positive thinking, all healing comes from the hand of the Divine Healer, God. His timing is perfect, and He is in control of all things.

I imagine fasting as having raised hands toward heaven, opening flesh and spirit to the healing power of God. Therefore, I praise God and thank the fast and paleo—all of which contributed to my healing.

Do your part and God will do the rest! If I found a solution after ten years, there's hope for you. Your healing is at hand.

Many others were healed on that fast as well. It's for
seek healing, so seek and you shall find!

Liver Cleansing: I also highly recommend liver cleanses.
This drink comes with the added benefit of flattening the
stomach!

4 cups of water

1 organic lemon, chopped

2 tablespoons of olive oil

Blend in mixer and drain. Add organic vanilla or ginger
for a delicious pop of flavor!

Bone Broth: How often do you read or hear advertisements
for medications to alleviate irritable bowel syndrome (IBS),
also referred to as leaky gut? My digestive issues were similar
to IBS, and after adding bone broth to my diet, my symptoms
went away within three months. Bone broth contains several
beneficial components that boost the immune system and
promote healing. Besides treating leaky gut syndrome, it can
also help you overcome food allergies and intolerances. You
may further notice an improvement in your joints, a reduction
in cellulite, and enhanced mental clarity.

Over the ages, doctors and mothers alike have prescribed
chicken soup for all kinds of illnesses. The warmth and flavor are
not only satisfying when you're under the weather, but all bone
broths — beef, chicken, fish, lamb, etc. — are easy to digest
and full of vital nutrients, including minerals. Of course, they
make great bases for all kinds of dishes, even the finest cuisine.
Perhaps that's why broths appear as staples in every culture.

The principle of not wasting any of the animal has existed
since ancient times. Boiling bones and marrow, as well as
tougher parts like ligaments to make them useful, comes with
the advantage of releasing powerful healing compounds, such
as collagen, proline, glycine, and glutamine.

You can thank the collagen for healing your gut lining, reducing intestinal inflammation, making your skin look and feel more youthful, and reducing the appearance of cellulite. If you're thinking more clearly, it's the glycine, which detoxifies your cells from chemicals and improves brain function.

I typically drink eight ounces upon waking every morning and recommend consuming eight ounces, one to two times daily. You could drink it plain as a beverage or add ingredients to make a soup. A bone broth fast also allows you to combine all the wonderful benefits of the broth and a fast.

Please reference the resource section in the back of the book to learn where to purchase grass-fed bones.

Other Nutrition Plans

Although paleo has worked for me, you may not want to choose that route. In that case, the goal is to select one of many other options that you'd enjoy. I'm not referring to a diet in the usual sense. Besides, who doesn't cringe upon hearing the d-word! It's time to be done with dieting! Instead, adjust your lifestyle to make healthier choices. I really want you to choose and live with foods you love.

By the way, my husband says I've become a much better cook now that I'm on paleo. Simply, I love the food.

Another route that appeals to many ladies now is the Mediterranean style of eating, traditionally followed in France, Italy, Greece, Spain, and Portugal—countries that have strikingly lower rates of cardiovascular disease compared to the U.S. The focus is on eating fish, whole grains, fresh fruits, fresh vegetables, legumes, nuts, and olive oil, and minimizing sugar, caffeine, junk food, and processed foods as much as possible.

Start with five servings of fruits and veggies every day. One serving equals four ounces, or about one-half cup. Be careful with fruit. I'd have severe swelling in my abdomen after eating fruit because of the sugar. Sugar also causes some to feel soreness in their joints from inflammation. Monitoring your reactions to foods will give you a feel for what works for your body. Fresh rather than canned or frozen—unless the whole, fresh food is flash-frozen—is always best, especially because processed foods generally contain sugar, salt, and other additives. When shopping, learn to read labels so that you can make the most nutritious choices.

Moreover, not all vegetables are equal. Cut way back on starchy ones, like potatoes and corn, in addition to white rice and anything made with white flour—including breads, muffins, bagels, biscuits, crackers, and pretzels. Such foods are all heavy in high-glycemic carbs, which too quickly raise blood sugar and insulin levels to high levels. High blood sugar and subsequent high insulin are two factors that cause your body to store fat. You don't have to eliminate high-glycemic carbs completely, but you should eat them in moderation. And when you do eat them, choose the healthiest version. A baked potato is healthier than French fries, for example, but, evidently, the woman at the McDonald's counter did not think so! Smile!

Special Note: About one in four women is gluten intolerant, especially after age fifty, and has far better digestion when avoiding wheat products. I definitely fall in this category. If you're having issues, get off gluten as a trial to see if eliminating it helps. You should feel better within two weeks, maybe earlier. Don't skimp on lean protein; it's an important part of any diet. Getting enough protein helps prevent carbohydrate cravings and increases glucagon, which jumpstarts your body into burning fat. Make sure that you eat protein with every meal and snack.

The healthiest source of animal protein is fish—especially mackerel, herring, salmon, trout, halibut, and fish canned in oil. The cold-water fish are high in heart-healthy omega-3 fats. Strive to have fish at least two or three times a week. Organic chicken and turkey are other good sources of animal protein for those who don't want fish. Lean cuts of beef—I prefer, and nutrition experts recommend, grass-fed, pasture-fed—and pork come next. Game meats, such as venison and buffalo, are also naturally lean and healthy. Other good sources of protein include organic eggs and dairy food. Raw, organic dairy products are the healthiest and most digestible because pasteurization destroys healthful enzymes.

Cutting way down on sweets, junk food, which turns to sugar in your body, and most processed food items is the most important thing you can do for several reasons. Besides the problem of sugar, processed foods, often containing unhealthy trans fats often found in cookies, crackers, and other snack foods, as well as in margarine and shortening, increase cellular inflammation. Inflammation keeps loading on the pounds.

Nitric Oxide: Unlike nitrous oxide, the gas that your dentist may use to calm you before a procedure, nitric oxide is a supplement you'll find advertised as a muscle enhancer for workouts. It's overall value to the body goes well beyond that.

Research from Harvard Medical School's Herbert Benson M.D., a scientific pioneer in the realm of mind-body medicine, shows that higher levels of nitric oxide molecules in the brain trigger yearnings that lead to profound spiritual experiences. The body naturally creates nitric oxide as a feel-good endorphin—a benefit to emotional and spiritual health. In other words, boosting nitric oxide helps the healing process, increases immunity, and works to prevent chronic degenerative diseases. Further, it keeps you physically strong and healthy as you age, improves your mood and outlook on life, and feeds your spirit and sense of belonging.

Dr. Northrup also suggests that nitric oxide, when released in the lining of the blood vessels, widens them to improve circulation throughout the body. Another plus is an increase in feel-good chemicals, such as serotonin and beta-endorphin, so the subconscious mind gets the message that you are happy, and an overall feeling of wellbeing is a side effect. Happier and calmer, your body functions more optimally and heals faster.

Living an extremely stressful lifestyle with minimal adventure or fun can deplete your nitric oxide levels. Therefore, you may want to take the supplement, but make sure your source does not contain soy.

Besides taking any supplements, seek and create joy in your life. All the while, keep working on your food choices until your plan works for you! Don't give up. This is an absolute must for you to be your best you!

Saltwater Tip: Add nitric oxide to your diet.

CHAPTER FOUR
Crashing Down

**"The cure for anything is salt water:
sweat, tears or the sea."
Isak Dinesen**

"I should have picked up on all the cues," Jacquelyn confessed, as we turned the corner on our morning walk. It was our last vacation together, and Larry's best friend met us at the beach house in Seaside."

Larry was Jacquelyn's former husband.

"His friend surprised us by dropping in and bringing his new girlfriend along," Jacquelyn continued. "She was twenty-six. I was cringing and covering my body much of the weekend. I'd already started putting on some weight. I guess that was Larry's subtle way of telling me he had similar plans up ahead. I feel so stupid! How did I miss all the signs? They were there, had I only looked."

Exasperated, Jacquelyn turned to me and said, "I'm ready to go deep; I'm ready to look up under the hood, as you call it, Victoria!"

We looked at our calendars and I blocked a two-hour session for her. We had lot of work ahead. Two hours would give us a jumpstart and undergird all that we needed to lay out. At that juncture, Larry had met a lady in her twenties and moved in with her. Somehow, the kids blamed it all on Jacquelyn, as if she were the sole bad guy. My heart ached for her, so I was delighted to have her joining me on walks. She had spent months depressed and sleeping after losing her business, her husband, and her kids' devotion.

It was all too much to bear. The bad stress in her life had soared through the roof, raising her cortisol levels as Jacquelyn's weight continued to escalate. She was barely hanging on in a battle to keep the mansion—her beautiful home where we'd had lunch and our tea time only two years prior. Her money was running out and she was desperate. Still, I smiled, knowing her commitment to therapy would take her to the beautiful life awaiting her on the other side.

Looking Under the Hood

On that first session of looking under the hood, we got cozy on the cushions in the room that I reserve in my home to see patients. To begin, I shared what God showed me on my morning walk.

We live near a lake, and I love taking nature walks through-out the year. During the spring and summer, the wildlife and gorgeous array of flowers, both planted and natural, and the old oak trees lift my spirits. In the South, a spring-like day can pop up in the middle of February as a surprise, although we know that March will return with frigid temperatures and high winds. Enjoying one of those gorgeous sneak previews of spring on that day in February, I was looking up to admire the crystal-clear sky, when my eye caught a bird's nest in a tree. It was a barren tree with no leaves and only a bird's nest in the branches. Although the tree and branches were entirely void of any protection, the nest was completely intact. As I continued my stroll, I saw nest after nest in barren trees. So many nests had survived the bulk of the harsh winter, and the birds were chirping. Breathing in the sunny rays and beautiful air, I wondered why I'd never noticed. After conveying my experience, I took a deep breath.

"Jacquelyn, this is a sign for you and me both! Yes, our nests are intact even after the winter storms. "Let's get started!"

And, so we began.

"Jacquelyn, I want to go way back," I calmly explained. "Tell me about your childhood and your family unit. I want to know as much detail as you can share. Don't hold back; the more you share, the more insight we will glean."

"Well," she replied, "I was raised in a wealthy family with a very dominant father and a mother who had a servant's heart. Everything hinged around my father's busy work schedule. He traveled, so when he was out of town, my three siblings and I would play with no restraints. Yet, when my father came home, it was all strict, straight laced, and no fun. He was such a disciplinarian—a very strong disciplinarian. I was the oldest and got the brunt of much of his discipline. He seemed always to try to blame me. When I would try to explain or fend for myself, he would cut me off. I always took the punishment for all the siblings. My voice was silenced. It was always father's way, no questions asked, what he says goes. I looked forward to his travels so that I could be expressive, play, and have fun. Secretly, I think my mother did, too!"

Jacquelyn went on for the entire two hours, which was typical. My first three sessions with a client are usually filled with the person talking and sharing. Listening enables me to recognize patterns. Eventually, I interject.

In one session, Jacquelyn shared a story of when she was older. She had been diligently working on a creative science fair project and received accolades from teachers at school. Most expected her to take first prize, and it mattered to Jacquelyn because she had put her heart into the work. One day before, however, her brother, one year younger than Jacquelyn, presented a similar display. The teachers and judges viewed projects from lower classmen to upperclassmen, and upon seeing her brother's first, they were so impressed that they awarded him first prize. Jacquelyn did not even place since her project was similar to a student's in a lower grade. Besides, it would have been awkward to give two first prizes to the same family. Only later did her brother confess that he'd stolen her idea.

At that point, she vowed to go after her heart's desire aggressively, not counting on anyone but herself. The betrayal from a family member, her own brother, stung deeply. It set the stage for her strong business drive, which ended up being both good and bad. She clothed herself with achieving and accomplishing on her own, not trusting anyone. She attracted another aggressive driver and they married. However, a big fault line of trust issues existed. It did not take too many sessions to understand that men had silenced her voice, stolen her dreams, and cut her off. No doubt, her husband joined the others in abandoning her.

The False Belief System

So often, because of life events, women create false beliefs to protect themselves. Unfortunately, those assumptions end up causing more harm than good. While possibly protective for a time, such as in childhood, a false belief system can block one's wellbeing. Letting go of it in adulthood is vital.

Jacquelyn's false belief system was becoming clear: If I express my true self I will be shut down.

She believed she'd be punished for expressing herself. In response, Jacquelyn tensed up and burrowed her way through college and the business world. Carrying a tough exterior and letting few people in, even though she was able to make it big in the business world, she developed a tough exterior and would not fully let people get in close.

Hero Story

Lee Rhodes, who was in her fifties when she founded Glassbaby, which makes handblown votives, overcame cancer three times. Something from the light from a votive gave her hope, which inspired her company. A portion of every sale is donated to causes that benefit humans, animals, and the environment. Her encouragement is to slow down and pay attention to what's important in life.

I'm honored that we became so close that she let me into her real and true heart issues. That is God's grace. If you are walking in a wounded state, be open to God's bringing a kindred-spirit into your life. Divine connections are priceless. Sharing from your heart with safe people has big rewards!

When I expressed Jacquelyn's false belief system aloud to her, she felt extreme anxiety. Her stress level was off the charts. She also told me that she felt sick at her stomach.

I knew what we needed to do next.

The Tapping Solution

As explained by Nick Ortner, author of the bestselling *The Tapping Solution*, therapeutic tapping is not the same as the tap-tap-tapping you'd enjoy while watching Gene Kelly and Debbie Reynolds tap-dancing in the musical *Singin' in the Rain*.

In the 1970s, Roger Callahan introduced the concept of tapping on specific areas of the body—endpoints of meridians on the body—to elicit a calming effect. Ortner says, "while focusing on the stress, the trauma, the anxiety, the pain, whatever's bothering us, we actually send a calming signal to the amygdala in the brain." Amygdala refer to the brain's "fight or flight" response center, the area that activates when someone experiences stress. Tapping neutralizes the amygdala. Ortner expresses that tapping sends a calming signal that "re-encodes" the memory rather than erasing it. "You still remember what happened," says Ortner, "but you have distance from it. The charge behind the memory is gone from it."

In my practice, I've found that tapping can be a wonderful way for individuals like Jacquelyn to manage extreme stress. I knew that her cortisol levels would have been off the charts with all she had going against her all at once.

If a similar feeling describes your situation, please have a doctor assess your cortisol levels and your hormonal levels.

The Stress Hormone: Cortisol

Your body has a built-in mechanism for protecting you from the effects of acute, immediate stress. If in the wild, you may experience the "stress response" upon seeing a tiger approach. Your adrenal gland would be busy producing several hormones, and the sudden "adrenaline rush" would give you the momentum to run away.

Likewise, whether facing the impending danger of a wild animal or feeling attacked by people and circumstances in your everyday life, you experience a vast release of cortisol, also known as the stress hormone. If in the wild, you'd run away from the tiger, thereby releasing your stress and feeling fine at some point upon reaching safety.

What happens if you don't find a way to escape your stressful situations and let it all go?

Chronic overexposure to cortisol can be devastating. When persistent, elevated cortisol in the body keeps blood sugar levels high, causes the bones to lose substantial levels of calcium, reduces the body's immune responses, raises blood pressure, leads to the loss of muscle mass, causes fat accumulation, and interferes with cognitive function.

A Powerful Weapon Against Anxiety: Rhodiola

Rhodiola is a natural, plant-based compound—an adaptogen—that enhances resistance to stress. Namely, it reduces harmful cortisol levels. Related benefits include improved sleep quality, boosted immunity, and restored vital organ function. From demonstrating restorative effects throughout the body in scientific studies, rhodiola potentially has the power to increase longevity and health. Evidence also shows that it minimizes depression and anxiety, improves cognitive function, increases muscle performance and endurance, prevents muscle damage, improves blood circulation, and burns fat. In Russia and Scandinavia, people have used rhodiola to alleviate everyday symptoms of anxiety and insomnia for centuries.

Hormone Basics

I'm grateful to Dr. Zoe Wells, N.D., who provided the in-depth descriptions of hormones and imbalances. Although the information is technical, it's important to know for you to communicate and pinpoint issues, and, therefore, could come in handy with future doctor visits.

What estrogen does in the body:

1) Supports elasticity in the tissue

2) Moisturizes and hydrates tissue, including skin

3) Keeps the bladder healthy

4) Supports a normal sleep cycle

5) Grants a feeling of emotional wellbeing

6) Makes the endometrium (lining of the uterus) grow, which is shed during the period when a woman is not pregnant

7) Supports hair growth

8) Makes the brain function and supports memory

9) Supports bone density

Though not as commonly talked about as estrogen, progesterone takes an active role with notable effects in the body. Progesterone is the hormone that allows the egg to be released each month during ovulation. After the egg release, the follicle makes more progesterone. Progesterone is typically the first hormone to change in perimenopause. When periods come closer together or further apart, progesterone is out of balance. If you don't ovulate or if you have ovarian cysts, you won't make as much progesterone, so you'll also likely suffer more PMS symptoms.

What progesterone does in the body:

1) Acts as an anti-inflammatory

2) Helps build bone

3) Calms the brain acting as an anti-anxiety agent

4) Supports normal sleep cycles

5) Regulates the period

6) Maintains fluid balance and water retention in the body

7) Supports orgasms

While the levels are lower in women than in men, testosterone is important for females.

What testosterone does in the body:

1) Strengthens tissue like the bladder and labia

2) Supports the libido or sex drive

3) Strengthens muscles

4) Provides physical endurance

5) Maintains bone density

Bioidentical hormones are hormones made in a lab that have the same chemical and physical structure as those made by the body. They differ from the synthetic hormones in birth control pills, which have a different biochemical structure from natural hormones.

Adrenal glands, located on the top of the kidneys, are crucial for the functioning of the body and the production of adrenal hormones. The adrenals produce cortisol, aldosterone, epinephrine, norepinephrine and the androgens: precursors to estrogen and testosterone.

The thyroid gland is in the neck and produces thyroid hormones that work in conjunction with the adrenals to affect energy levels as well as the energy needed to run each cell in the body. The thyroid is the body temperature and cellular function regulator, affecting fat burning, cellular repair, cholesterol metabolism, and serum calcium balance.

Symptoms of Hormones Gone Awry

Hormones interact with one another in an intricate and complex fashion. When all hormones are produced and secrete normally, the glands communicate amicably and support one another in maintaining hormonal balance and well-being. The brain receives the feedback message that all is well; this is homeostasis.

Compare your hormones to a beautiful symphony. The performance melts your heart when all notes and instruments are in sync. If someone hit the wrong note or goes flat in the delivery, the result is unpleasant to hear and possibly downright embarrassing for the musician. Similarly, even when one hormone becomes imbalanced, all the other hormones downstream are affected. The brain gets the message that a problem has occurred, so the pituitary and hypothalamus respond by sending out further signals, or chemical messages, to the glands to fix the problem.

With either too much or too little of specific hormones, symptoms such as these may occur:

- Estrogen Imbalance
- Excess weight that won't come off
- Depression
- Sleep problems, insomnia
- Poor memory, a foggy head and problems thinking clearly
- Hair loss
- Dry skin, increased wrinkles
- Vaginal dryness
- Pain with intercourse

- Hot flashes
- Bladder infections
- Progesterone Imbalance
- Anxiety, worry
- Heart palpitations
- Problems sleeping especially waking during the night
- Hot flashes and night sweats
- Panic attacks
- Water retention
- Breast tenderness

- Difficulty having an orgasm
- Testosterone Imbalance
- Weakness
- Poor physical stamina
- Low libido

- Incontinence
- Weight gain around middle
- Acne
- Increased facial hair growth

Adrenal symptoms:

- Lightheaded, disoriented
- Low blood sugar
- Low blood pressure
- Fatigue
- Difficulty waking in morning
- Nervousness, anxiety
- A sense of being wired and tired
- Feeling stressed, overreacting to stress, inability to cope with stress

- Thyroid Symptoms
- Hair loss or thinning
- Dry skin
- Fatigue, tiredness
- Depression
- Wanting excess sleep
- Cold body temperature
- Loss of outer 1/3 of eyebrows
- Constipation

Assessing Hormone Status

As you can see, hormonal balance is crucial to well-being. I recommend working with a practitioner who can assess your hormone status and provide you with treatment to bring hormones back into balance. The process, however, is not straightforward. While having the list will assist in highlighting your issues, be prepared for your symptoms to change as you progress through perimenopause. Your awareness allows you to stay on top of the changes.

According to Dr. Zoe Wells, ND, practitioners vary widely in their experience and expertise in hormone or endocrine function. You must choose a practitioner who is up to date and well versed in endocrine issues. When selecting a professional to guide you, ask each what kind of lab work they use to assess hormones and how they treat endocrine issues. The most experienced practitioners will use saliva or blood tests to measure hormones, and some will use twenty-four-hour urine tests. Cortisol is best tested in saliva, whereas the other hormones can be tested in either blood, saliva, or urine.

Find a doctor who will test for the following hormones for each of the endocrine glands:

estradiol, estrone, progesterone, testosterone (total and free), DHEA-sulfate, cortisol, thyroid-stimulating hormone (TSH) free, triiodothyronine (T3) free, thyroxine (T4), and anti-thyroid antibodies

Importantly, slow down and pay attention. Writing your observations down will help. Having a history of your physical shifts and changes helps to demonstrate the hormonal flux and what needs to be brought back into balance. This approach can help your doctor in his or her assessments.

Back to Jacquelyn

Jacquelyn added nitric oxide and rhodiola rosea to her supplements. She is also under the care of a medical doctor who is monitoring her health and following her blood work as she makes a few shifts with supplements. Together, we are working to lower her cortisol levels and get her hormones into balance.

Also, as her tears began flowing freely, Jacquelyn started the healing process. She's now moving, walking, and sweating, all the while looking at the hard issues and false beliefs. Despite many tears, her tapping and new supplements have helped her tremendously as her hormones shift.

As the Danish author Isak Dinesen (1885 – 1962) said, "The cure for anything is salt water: sweat, tears or the sea!"

Saltwater Tip: Two powerful tools to lower stress and cortisol levels are rhodiola and tapping.

Get moving and sweating. Look under the hood to locate those old, false and limiting beliefs, and heal them with as many tears as you need. Why not take a vacation to an idyllic spot on the beach? You deserve it you—really!

I'm so delighted to be sharing with you, but can we stop, right now, for a moment? Put this book down, look yourself in the mirror and say:

I love, honor and respect myself!

Now, give yourself a big hug. You are a beautiful lady! Ready now? Let's continue on this journey!

DISCLAIMER: I am not a medical doctor. I do not recommend that you take any supplements or make any changes without checking with your physician and/ or natural practitioner. I do recommend that you have a trusted professional monitor you carefully if and as you add any supplement.

FREE GIFT: 19 Ways to Improve Your Relationships
Increase your passion. Gain and establish trust.
Enjoy the love you've always wanted.
GO TO FindingHeavenBook.com/pages/bonus

CHAPTER FIVE

Overcoming Gossip and Cliques

**"When people show you who they are,
believe them the first time."
Maya Angelou**

As I entered my home, arms and hands full of grocery bags, my cell phone was ringing. Dropping some of my bags on the floor, I glanced at it and saw that Shani had called three times. Oh, no. Something was wrong. I listened to her message, and Shani's voice was upset. Some toxic ordeal had gone down—something about the theatre where she worked. The rest of the message was garbled. I took a deep breath. I really did not want to get involved, but I decided to carve out some time for her. Her mother had recently passed away, and she possibly needed a listening, caring ear.

Shani's passion for the theatre began at an early age. A student of voice, she had attended a special arts high school before winning a scholarship to Juilliard and majoring in theatre with a minor in voice. She performed Off-Broadway, where she met her husband and moved back to Atlanta to raise their children. Shani was overqualified to direct for a community theatre group, but her love of kids and musicals prompted her to take on the role. I respected Shani very much. She easily could have been in another setting being paid considerably more money. Our group of friends had encouraged her to send a script to Eugene Wisenburg for an Off-Broadway production, and as negotiations were underway, we were all secretly praying for her success. Shani had blessed so many, and this could be her big break!

I called her back and she answered.

"I've been fired!" she choked out between sobs. "I can't believe it. I've been fired!"

I was speechless because Shani, in the view of many, was the most talented and creative director in town and had been directing for years. People would come from all over to see her musicals. Everyone knew she was overqualified for her position. On top of that, if your child got picked for a lead, you knew she or he had real talent!

"Guess who?" Shani continued.

"Oh, no," I said. "Don't tell me. Please don't tell me any names."

"Elizabeth St. James!" she blurted out.

Now that the cat was out of the bag, I responded, "Really? She's still involved at the theatre?"

"Oh, yes," Shani replied, "and her daughter is a senior this year. That's what stirred up all the trouble."

Everyone knew Elizabeth St. James was from old money. She was also politically active and socially connected. She knew all the right people. A trophy wife, Elizabeth was a gorgeous woman, but something within her core was terribly wrong. She was as mean as a snake. She loved to gossip, and she loved having power over people. She was a woman who was used to getting her way. She had quite the reputation. Newcomers learned the hard way after falling on her bad side. A few well-placed words could have you out on your ear. Everyone tipped-toed around her to stay on her good side. Shani made the misfortunate mistake of being too much of a professional in her job.

Elizabeth knew that her daughter Ashley, a high school senior, could not reach the high notes, but she was certain her child would receive the leading role. What talent cannot bring, donations can. The board of directors at the theatre loved Elizabeth; she greased their palms with lots of dough.

"Another younger girl, a sophomore, just blew us away during the auditions," Shani told me. "We went with her for the lead. I guess I should have seen it all coming down the pike, but I did not notice. I was too busy directing and pulling each act together. The show was flawless! Standing ovations for each performance. As we were busy with the production and rehearsals, from what I can tell, Elizabeth St. James had an entire entourage stirred up against me."

My eyes snapped back to my grocery bags on the floor in the foyer. Out of the corner of my eye, I saw Lulu, one of my three, gorgeous Australian Shepherds, or Aussies, acting strangely. Lulu was always my spitfire ball of energy, but she was lethargically sprawled over the arm of the couch in the living room.

"Shani," I said. "I need to go. Come over here later this afternoon, if you can, and let's see if we can unpack this."

Wondering about Lulu, I went about the business of collecting the grocery bags I'd left in the foyer. That's when I noticed a paper tray on the floor. As soon as I picked it up, I realized it was the tray from the bottom of a rotisserie chicken.

"LuLu!" I screamed! "Where's the chicken? Where's . . . the . . . chicken! Oh, I can't believe she ate the whole thing!"

My forty-pound Aussie had wolfed down an entire rotisserie chicken while I had been on my call!

Terrified, I called my vet. He said to give her bread—lots of bread. Surprisingly, while she lay there moaning, she still managed to eat the bread! The vet said to watch her carefully for any strange behavior or gagging motions, but he was happy it was a rotisserie chicken. They are cooked long enough to soften the bones, making them easier to digest. Thankfully, Lulu lounged around for about three hours and then was her spunky active self again.

These Aussies are my babies. I highly recommend doggies while making the menopausal passage! They are the most unconditionally loving sweethearts in the world. Anyone else a doggie lover? Yes, I know you are! Smile!

I was throwing a ball to my Aussies when Shani drove up the driveway for her session. When I greeted her, the tears were already flowing down her cheeks. I grabbed a tissue box for her, and we curled up on pillows in my upstairs office. I love having my office in my home because it's so intimate and warm. Creating such an environment is a beautiful way to nurture kindred spirits and caring hearts.

Shani had been working on her spiritual side by getting still and taking time to hear from God. She had been part of the group who had participated in the powerful, twenty-one-day fast. That miraculous experience alone had made a huge impression on us all—one we would not forget. It certainly seemed that God had been undergirding Shani with his love and preparing her heart for this nasty storm a blowin' in.

"They've let me go," Shani said. Drying her tears, she was still sniffling and taking deep breaths. "The same week Momma passed away, I was called into the office at the theatre. And they've let me go."

"What happened?"

I took a deep breath. I was trying to maintain my composure and objectivity. At times like this, that's a little harder than you can imagine.

"Well, as you know," she continued, "Momma passed away, and one of the ladies from the theatre drove me to the airport. I thought she was acting a little strangely. My perception was correct. We had just finished our musical. The show was flawless! I had picked the children who really had the talent and were perfect for each part. Standing ovations for each performance. As we were busy with the production and rehearsals, Elizabeth, the woman whose daughter did not get the lead, became very busy gossiping. Her daughter had talent and was in her senior year; however, another younger girl, a sophomore, just blew us away during the auditions. We went with the younger girl for the lead. Like I said, Elizabeth's daughter had talent, but just could not hit those high notes. I have to take the entire production into consideration. I guess I should have seen it all coming down the pike, but I was concentrating on pulling the talent out of these kids, act by act."

"From what I could tell," Shani continued, "before it was said and done, Elizabeth had a loyal circle of friends spreading gossip throughout the community. Most of them were board members for the theatre and moms who had children in the production. Anyone from the outside could have seen through this but not the inner clique that formed."

Gossip is one of those strange entities that forms a life of its own.

Once the gossip and perceived offenses started, a toxic and touchy group flared up against Shani. The most unfortunate part was that it all came to a head the week her mother passed away.

"They ran me out on a rail!" Shani cried out and burst into tears. "Also, Eugene Wisenburg called, and they've changed their minds about my script. They've decided to go with another writer/director." More sobs erupted from her.

Silently, I was praying, Dear God, why is all this turmoil blowing in on sweet, precious Shani? Please, stop the storms. My mother's heart just wanted to wrap her up in a blanket and rock her. I knew this was a toxic setup, straight from the pit of hell. We had lots of work to do. Not only was she grieving her mother's passing, but also had the unjust firing and disappointment regarding her script piled on top.

Shani said that women who had loved her throughout the years turned on her. It was as if she had never seen those sides to them. This behavior was shocking to say the least. Many were on the board of directors for the theatre, and those ladies had raved about Shani and her productions for many years. Shani had an amazing track record for sold-out productions.

I let Shani get it all out, a process that took more than several sessions. When someone is grieving a deep loss, we go slowly and allow for grieving. We were at the point to start some healing exercises when I received another call from Shani.

Elizabeth St. James wanted to meet her for lunch. Shani was hopeful there would be apologies and they could put the entire mess behind them. I had my hunch that the lunch would not go quite that smoothly. Shani, always seeing the best in others, felt differently, so I warned her to be careful and use discernment with her conversation.

I reminded her of Maya Angelou's quote: "When people show you who they are, believe them the first time."

Shani met Elizabeth at an upscale restaurant with a lovely view the shore of the Chattahoochee River. Sitting next to the window, Elizabeth was pleasant enough to the waiter before orchestrating what would transpire next.

"Shani, my darlin'," Elizabeth said, emphasizing her Southern drawl, "please tell me how your children are doing?"

The chitchat seemed innocent enough, but Elizabeth's tone soon changed.

"You know, Shani, I was at a party the other night, and one of my dear friends, Eugene Wisenburg, and I were talking, he thought that he might know you."

Shani sat up quickly. "Why, yes, I do know him," Shani said.

"Well, I just told him you were directing our children's play," Elizabeth continued. "I had no idea you were going for anything beyond community theatre. When Eugene and I made the connection that we both mutually knew you, I said, 'You couldn't possibly be considering Shani for Off-Broadway, she's just a cheap hack, and the only reason we have her is she's the only one who would direct our children for free!'"

Elizabeth let out an evil chuckle.

Shocked, Shani stammered, "What . . . what else did you say to him?"

"Oh, only that you directed our children's theatre," Elizabeth replied in her haughty tone.

"Well, what was his response?" Shani couldn't stop herself from asking.

"Oh, honestly, Shani! It was just a passing connection, and I really don't remember."

This was the knife that Elizabeth twisted into Shani's heart. Shani became flushed and excused herself to the restroom. Splashing some cool water on her face, she was determined to maintain her composure until she could exit the restaurant. All the while, Elizabeth sat at the table, gloating over her thoughts about her conversation with Eugene Wisenburg:

Eugene: *Isn't your daughter involved in a musical? What part did she get?*

Elizabeth: *Well, she should have got the lead, but we have a subpar director for this play. Shani just has no talent.*

Eugene: *Shani, that's an unusual name. What's her last name?*

They made the connection.

Elizabeth: *You can't be considering a housewife with so little talent. She directs children's theatre. Why, Eugene, I'm surprised at you! You'd be a laughing stock to go with Shani. They would chase you out of Manhattan!*

Elizabeth wore a cat-who-swallowed-the-birdie grin when Shani returned. Sitting, yet squirming for an exit plan, she let Elizabeth talk.

"Well, Shani, I wanted to bring you here and talk to you personally because we are friends. As you know I'm on the board of directors for the theatre, and I'm sorry to inform you that you've been voted out by other members of the board for next year's musical as well. Many donors feel that the play this year just did not go in the direction they wanted, and they would like to bring in fresh talent. Namely, they want Haden Bloom to take over as director. Of course, next year, you will be able to stay on and help, but all directing decisions will be made by Haden from this point on."

Feeling a wave of nausea, Shani thought she'd pass out. Something was literally sucking the life out of her. Little else of Elizabeth's monologue registered, but Shani remembered hearing that somehow the kindness bestowed on her should be a big favor considering her mother's passing. She would be relieved of a heavy load to bear!

Elizabeth sat with a devilish grin as she slaughtered Shani, blow by blow. Escaping again to the restroom, Shani managed to pull her thoughts together, close out her tab, and ran to her car before sobbing. She sobbed so hysterically on the way home that she had to pull over on the side of the road.

The event was so traumatic for Shani that it overloaded her emotions beyond the point she could process.

When a person goes through deep trauma and the emotions are too much to handle, sometimes his or her brain will freeze-frame the event. Painful memories associated with the trauma stay frozen until it's safe to let them thaw out. Shani had enough with her mother passing, the drama group turning against her, losing her job as director, and finally hearing that Elizabeth had manipulated the situation that cost her the Off-Broadway deal.

Can we all sit back and say, "Evil woman!" What would cause a person to be so mean?

You guessed it! Elizabeth St. James is a narcissist. The fact that she did not get her way, enabling her daughter to play the lead role, wounded Elizabeth's ego to the point of spending the better part of a year to undermine every single piece of Shani's life that she could manipulate. Wow!

I had to educate Shani on the differences between a toxic person and a toxic group. Investing in just one toxic person can be more than taxing and have a horrible effect on our physical and emotional wellbeing. Hopefully, we find some space and a reprieve from the one person. When it's a group, we have the intensity of "group act." People in a toxic group are more likely to behave in toxic ways, even when it's not consistent with their own individual behavior. When we experience this, we feel like everyone is against us.

Oftentimes, it's one toxic person who spearheaded and stirred the group into a toxic cocktail! Usually, the person is wounded and hurting.

In Shani's situation, one intensely hurtful wound came from Allana, one of the women who had joined the fast with us. The two would often get together and pray over the children and the productions. Unfortunately, Allana had been blindsided by the group and joined the gossipy mix. Shani was left unsure of who was with her and was not. Friend or foe, she could not decipher.

I was so saddened that Shani had the experience; however, I knew that God was calling her to a very high place. It was a classic case of a queen bee and her wanna bees stirring up trouble in the hive.

If you have ever been burned by a narcissist, you understand the lengths such a person will go. Well, it took Shani and me some time to put the pieces together, yet we finally figured out what had been missing from the puzzle.

Some people never outgrow the egocentric childhood belief that their needs are the only important ones, and the related traits of narcissism and self-absorption certainly seem prevalent these days. Lacking empathy and genuine interest in others, they grow into adults with a sense of bold superiority and a desire for respect and admiration from others, yet they offer little in return. Additionally, if events do not unfold as they expect, these people can become erratic and rude, often lashing out when criticized.

According to narcissism expert Dan Neuharth, PhD, also a licensed marriage and family therapist in the San Francisco Bay Area, "As we grow, most of us learn that we aren't the center of the universe, that other people have legitimate feelings and needs, and that we can't always get what we want. Developmentally, narcissistic and self-absorbed people haven't yet accepted these realities or their limitations and therefore often respond to frustrations with a child's repertoire: sulking, blaming, avoiding, manipulating, throwing a tantrum or acting out in other ways."

Dr. Neuharth explains that narcissists "live and operate in a different world," so establishing "healthy boundaries" is fundamental to preventing them from causing harm. The following has been shared by Dr. Neuharth, PhD. MFT, in *Narcissism Decoded*:

1. View them with compassion. It may not be easy to be sympathetic, but it may be better for your own emotional health. Contrary to popular belief that narcissism is extreme self-esteem, it can actually stem from fear, insecurity and lack of self-esteem.

"Underneath their self-centeredness, they are likely afraid of feeling flawed, powerless, unworthy or out of control," says Neuharth. "Knowing this may enable you to take their actions less personally."

2. But don't let them take advantage. Narcissistic and self-absorbed people are good at getting what they want,

and you may find yourself always in the path of their needs.

"If someone is repeatedly focusing on what you can do for them, you have the right to say no or tell them you will think about it and get back to them," Neuharth says.

"If someone is being pushy or critical, it can help to have assertive phrases ready such as, 'I am satisfied I did the right thing,' or, 'I will consider your ideas as well as mine.'"

3. Shield yourself emotionally. Since the narcissist in your life will likely think his/her ideas and approach are better than yours, prepare yourself for pushback if you disagree or share an opinion; the other's point of view is so firmly entrenched in the I-am-right position.

"It may be a mistake to discuss personal matters," says Neuharth. "You may be vulnerable to ridicule or being dismissed."

Getting a meaningful dialog going is also unlikely—unless you agree with them.

4. Choose your reaction. It's easy to get aggravated around self-obsessed people but changing your expectation and realizing that narcissists don't have the same flexibility as you to step outside of their own way of seeing the world are also wise perspectives. Sometimes you must humor them and play along to keep the peace, for example, if the narcissist is your boss. Sometimes you can listen politely and move on. If in a relationship that is so slanted toward the needs of the other person, you sometimes have to pull away and observe behavior rather than react.

5. Stop giving so much. Relationships with narcissists and self-absorbed people can be one-way streets, but you can learn to not give in to selfish behavior.

"If you keep giving to someone who only takes and doesn't appreciate what you are giving, you are teaching them to be a taker, not a giver," says Neuharth.

Whether a friend is asking you once again to put your life on hold to help with something or an uncle is dominating every family dinner with his opinions and doesn't let you get in a word, you may decide to do less, give less, or spend less time catering to that individual. Although taking such a stance is difficult, you should stop enabling the behavior, at least while the person is around you, so you can focus on your own needs.

6. Make yourself a priority. Narcissists and self-absorbed people believe the world revolves around them; they are interested in you insofar as you are revolving around them, too. You, perhaps, would never think to tend to your own needs before the needs of other people the way a narcissist does.

"If you're not taking care of yourself, you will eventually have nothing to give and nothing to show for it except resentment," says Neuharth. "Healthy self-care means boundary-setting."

Also, after such a difficult situation, judging those who've caused great pain is natural. Be careful. Already hurt and rejected, you could easily pick up judgement as a great protector.

Seeking safety and protection, you want to judge back. I'll give an analogy of what this judgement cycle looks like on our souls.

Hero Story

Savona Bailey-McClain, founder and executive director of the West Harlem Art Fund, Inc., exposes the public to art and culture by presenting it in open venues. The organization also fosters opportunities for artists by showcasing their work. In her fifties, Savona loves her position, which allows her to travel and meet people.

71

When my children were younger, I would help with their science fair projects. Before the evening was up, the kids would be messing around with the glue and glitter and supplies. One evening, I had only two poster boards with both children each needing one, and my son had glued the two together. Both needed a poster board that night! As I tried so hard to pull them gently apart, no way were those boards coming unglued without pieces ripping and sticking.

What a picture of our souls and hearts being intertwined in judgement!

If we tend to it quickly, while the glue is still wet, we have a chance to pull the two apart. The longer we wait, the glue sets and the more difficult the task becomes.

Likewise, judging those who have hurt us causes their junk to stick to us. The longer we stew over the events and judge them, the more likely they are to stay stuck on us. The longer we wait, the harder it becomes to become unstuck.

How do we get unstuck and release them? Forgiveness is the answer. However, forgiveness has a process.

Saltwater Tip: Forgiveness comes upon taking each of five vital steps.

1. Be brave enough to look at the wound. Acknowledge and honor your hurt.

2. Recognize the judgements you are making because of the hurt.

3. See the person who hurt you as wounded to speed up healing and help you to glean compassion.

4. Pray for guidance from God to truly see the person who hurt you through the eyes of love. Put on spiritual eyes after being hurt. This, the hardest step, is a supernatural act of God.

5. Forgive.

The Shift to Forgiveness

Notice the shift. After you see the person with compassion, you can shift into forgiveness. Seeing the person who hurt you through eyes of love gives you permission to heal and let go.

I lay out the five steps as if this were a simple process. It's not. However, after we start the journey and seek God's guidance, He meets us in the midst of our healing. The key is clinging to God and spiritual guidance. I strongly believe it takes the supernatural to move through betrayals, offense and judgements.

Step One: Be brave enough to look at the wound.

Shani was able to complete the first step. She was brave enough to say, "Ouch! This hurts deeply!" Surprisingly, many stay stuck right here on pride. They live in denial that they were hurt, yet they spew out more rejection, gossip, criticism, and judgements, which, in return, come back to hurt them deeply. It's a boomerang of hurt: you've already been hurt, so now you are hurting others.

You've possibly heard the saying, wounded people wound others. Let's take responsibility and get these wounds healed. When I hear someone gossiping, and it's a pattern for them, I know the person has deep, deep wounds that he or she has not dealt with yet.

With healing comes blessing and release. The Bible says, "The entire Law is fulfilled in a single decree: 'Love your neighbor as yourself.' But if you keep on biting and devouring each other, watch out, or you will be consumed by each other." Galatians 5:14,15.

Love of self and others is the key. Let's boomerang the love! When it's a boomerang blessing, everyone benefits. Shani was able to see that several of the mothers in the drama group were hurting. Elizabeth's actions left the entire group wounded. As a result, each one in the entire group was wounding Shani.

73

That's what a classic narcissist will do. Shani embraced that she was wounded deeply. Anger came up, yet she was more hurt than any other emotion. As she embraced the hurt, the tears were quite healing.

Let's drop our pride and embrace the wound. This huge step is critical in the healing process. Shani easily forgave the women in the drama group, but the wounds from Elizabeth struck a deeper cord. It would take some real spiritual heart surgery to remove the wound. Also, Allana was a closer connection and a prayer partner, so the hurt she caused went a little deeper as well. The closer the person is to you, the deeper the wound. Be aware of deeper wounds but realize that you can heal from them, too, in time.

Step Two: Recognize the judgements you are making because of the hurt.

This step was more difficult for Shani. She continued to rehearse over and over, "Why did Elizabeth do this!" "Allana, how dare she; we were close friends!" "How did she glean so much power against me?"

Making the betrayal so difficult was that it was imprinted in her mind around a separate traumatic event: her mother's passing. She was experiencing extreme sadness over a huge loss when the horrible news of losing her director's position and the deal with the Off-Broadway script going awry pushed right up against the death. The imprint of the three events together worked against Shani, causing a terribly bad cortisol reaction.

While grieving over her mother, she continued to stew over and over the events that led up to her being fired. Her sleeping patterns were disrupted. She grabbed at food for energy. Exhaustion kicked in, zapping her system, creating an energy leak.

I introduced Shani to Emotional Freedom Technique (EFT), referred to as Tapping. I learned the technique from Nick and Jessica Ortner's event, The Tapping Summit. The

Tapping script I use is from the interview Jessica Ortner conducted with Gabby Bernstein at The Tapping Summit.

EFT can be described as a psychological acupressure technique that supports your emotional health. More than five thousand years ago, the Chinese recognized a series of energy circuits that run through the body. The circuits, identified by the Chinese as meridians, are the bases for acupuncture and acupressure.

You can stimulate certain meridian points on your own body by tapping with your fingertips. In turn, you can release EFT's benefits, which, like acupuncture, include restoring energy and healing emotions.

When you tap on specific energy meridians found on your face, head, arm, and chest, you can release old fears, limiting beliefs, negative patterns, and even physical pain. While you tap, you talk out loud about the issue you are working to heal. Allowing yourself to speak and feel the emotions while simultaneously tapping on the energy points sends a signal to the brain that it's safe to relax.

The amygdala, located in the temporal lobes of the brain, release cortisol when you are in fight or flight mode. Cortisol levels remain elevated if the amygdala continue to fire and release long after the traumatic event has passed. EFT is a relaxing technique that signals the amygdala to quit firing the cortisol, as if saying, okay, you can relax now. From a relaxed state of being, you can process hurtful information, all of which promotes healing.

Emotional Freedom Technique (EFT) or Tapping: How It Works

Whenever you begin the tapping process, start with the Most Pressing Issue, or MPI. In Shani's case, the MPI was related to judgment. She started with the phrase, "I can't stop judging this person." The "person" may be one individual, a group of people, or even you. (You can modify the script below to best suit your situation.)

Next, rate your pre-tapping MPI on a scale of zero to ten, ten being the most distressing.

The process entails saying each line aloud while tapping on the corresponding meridian point. You can tap with either hand. You can also choose either side of your face or body on which to tap. The script guides you through a few rounds—referred to as negative rounds—in which you'll honor your fear, resentment, and discomfort.

As you start to feel a little relief from the negative rounds, you'll move into positive rounds by shifting the patterns around those thoughts. The shift from negative to positive will feel great. Your body will relax, your breath will deepen, and you will let go of the stressed-out trigger that has been releasing the bad cortisol.

Use the script below and tap on the designated areas of your body (meridian points) as you say the suggested phrases. Before you begin, review each meridian point in the image.

Tapping for Rejection from Betrayal

Rate your MPI. Ask yourself how emotionally charged you are when you think about the person who hurt you deeply and that you are now judging. Remember, the person can be a group or even yourself. You can replace the words "this person" with a name. Rate your MPI from zero to ten, ten being the most emotionally charged. Shani's MPI was ten-plus!

Tap on the karate chop point, as seen in the illustration, with your other hand. While tapping, repeat your phrase aloud three times. The following was Shani's script:

While tapping on the karate chop point: *Even though I can't stop judging Elizabeth and this drama group, I deeply and completely love and accept myself.*

76

Tapping Points

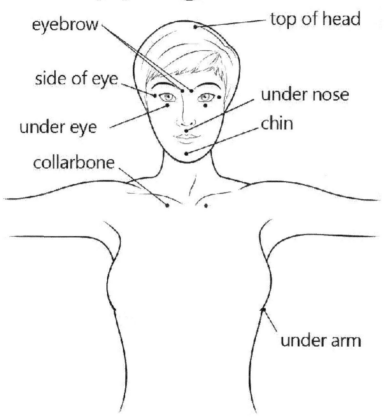

eyebrow

top of head

side of eye

under nose

under eye

chin

collarbone

under arm

While tapping on the karate chop point: *Even though I can't stop judging Elizabeth and this drama group, I deeply and completely love and accept myself.*

While tapping on the karate chop point: *Even though I can't stop judging Elizabeth and the moms of this drama group, I deeply and completely love and accept myself.*

While tapping on the karate chop point: *Even though I can't stop judging this drama group, I deeply and completely love and accept myself.*

Continue lightly tapping on the other meridians, one by one, while saying each phrase aloud.

Follow the sequence here:

Tapping on the eyebrow: I can't stop judging.

Tapping on the side of the eye: It feels so good to judge them.

Tapping under the eye: Judging makes me feel better about myself.

Tapping under the nose: And Elizabeth really deserves my judgment.

Tapping on the chin: They've done so much to make me want to judge.

Tapping on the collarbone: They deserve it, after all.

Tapping under the arm: I feel justified in my judgment.

Tapping on top of the head: Elizabeth deserves it!

Tapping on the eyebrow: If I give up judgment, I will be giving in.

Tapping on the side of the eye: I don't want to stop judging.

Tapping under the eye: Judging makes me feel better about myself.

Tapping under the nose: I believe I deserve to judge them for this.

Tapping on the chin: They've made me really upset.

Tapping on the collarbone: They've really gotten under my skin.

Tapping under the arm: They deserve it!

Tapping on top of the head: They deserve it!

Tapping on the eyebrow: They've upset me so much!

Tapping on the side of the eye: I deserve to judge them for what they've done.

Tapping under the eye: I just can't let it go.

Tapping under the nose: How could someone be that way?

Tapping on the chin: I'm so triggered by them.

Tapping on the collarbone: I'm so annoyed.

Tapping under the arm: I'm so aggravated by them.

Tapping on top of the head: They deserve it!

Tapping on the eyebrow: All this judgment.

Tapping on the side of the eye: I feel it's justified after all they've done.

Tapping under the eye: I have so many reasons to judge this person.

Tapping under the nose: It feels good to judge them.

Tapping on the chin: I feel safe when I judge them.

Tapping on the collarbone: I judge to protect myself.

Tapping under the arm: I need to do that because deep down I feel shame.

Tapping on top of the head: I want to heal my shame.

Tapping on the eyebrow: All this shame.

Tapping on the side of the eye: I don't even want to acknowledge it.

Tapping under the eye: I have to judge to avoid this shame.

Now shift to the positive:

Tapping under the arm: But I want to release it.

Tapping on top of the head: I want to heal so I can stop judging.

Continue to tap through the negative rounds outlined above. The moment you feel a sense of relief, you can begin the positive rounds:

Tapping on the eyebrow: But judgment doesn't really make me feel better.

Tapping on the side of the eye: Love actually makes me feel a lot better.

Tapping under the eye: But judging just seems easier.

Tapping under the nose: It feels safer to judge.

Tapping on the chin: I'm afraid of my shame, so I judge.

Tapping on the collarbone: I'm afraid of my shame.

Tapping under the nose: If I released judgment, who would I be?

Tapping on the chin: I guess I'd be left with me.

Tapping on the collarbone: Being me may be better.

Tapping under the arm: I have to release judgment to love myself again.

Tapping on the top of the head: If I release them, I will be free.

Tapping on the eyebrow: All the energy I spend judging could be spent on feeling good.

Tapping on the side of the eye: I could use the energy more wisely.

Tapping under the eye: And I could increase my energy by choosing to love rather than judge.

Tapping under the nose: I can also see that I'm judging a person who is in pain.

Tapping under the chin: I can see them with compassion.

Tapping on the collarbone: I can see that they're in pain.

Tapping under the arm: I want to send them love and prayers.

Tapping on top of the head: They just want to be happy. Just like me.

Tapping on the eyebrow: I want to be happy.

Tapping on the side of the eye: Releasing judgment sets me free to be happy.

Tapping under the eye: I'd much rather feel free.

Tapping under the nose: I choose to send love to this person.

Tapping on the chin: That love will clear my blocks.

Tapping on the collarbone: And I will feel that freedom.

Tapping under the arm: I choose love.

Tapping on top of the head: I choose to be free from judgment.

Tapping on the eyebrow: I want to be happy and free.

Tapping on the side of the eye: I want to forgive so I can feel good.

Tapping under the eye: I don't want to feel judgmental anymore.

Tapping under the nose: I pray for this person to feel good too.

Tapping on the chin: That love will clear my blocks.

Tapping on the collarbone: All I want is happiness.

Tapping under the arm: I choose happiness.

Tapping on the top of the head: I choose to be free from judgment.

Continue tapping through the positive statements as many times as you'd like until you feel genuine relief. When you're done, say your MPI out loud: "I can't stop judging this person."

Now rate it from zero to ten and compare your rating to when you first began. If you tapped through each round with commitment, you're sure to have experienced relief. In some cases, you may drop from a ten to a two in just a minute of tapping, although any relief is a miracle.

Shani's MPI dropped to a five. She had to continue tapping when she felt the stress. Each time she tapped, she experienced more freedom towards her full breakthrough.

After tapping for a couple of weeks, Shani was able to relax and move forward. Not only did she relax, but she also slept better, which helped her energy levels. She also quit grabbing at all the snacks to make it through the day. A doctor's appointment confirmed that her cortisol levels were coming down. Amazing! If you are stuck and your physical body is suffering, I wholeheartedly recommend tapping to enhance and speed up healing.

Step Three: See the person who hurt you as wounded to speed up healing and help you to glean compassion.
This step came quickly for Shani, as she gleaned more information from a friend who had been connected to the drama group but not in it. Many loved Shani. They knew exactly what was going on, and many in the community were grieved. Also, Shani did her homework regarding how to deal with

a narcissist and began learning how to set firm boundaries. The people-pleasing side to Shani was growing and learning.

God will give us the information we need to heal.

It's amazing how God will give you the information you need to heal. If you will be still and do your part, God comes in and provides the rest.

Quickly, Shani began to see the ladies as wounded, and before long, her caring, kind heart kicked in with the gift of mercy. Step three is a big shift. I've seen tragic situations in which this would seem impossible.

In one case, I counseled a young lady who had been raped. For her, we started by gathering information that she learned from the experience. Gathering information was a step in the right direction until she could view the person as one with a deeply wounded soul and a victim. I was so proud of her. This young lady ended up facing her rapist at the court case and forgiving him. Confessing that it had been a supernatural act of God for her to be able to forgive, she was able to see that he was a disturbed young man with no solid upbringing. His circumstances propelled him to wound others deeply. Shifting to see her perpetrator from that perspective took great courage, and she benefitted more than anyone.

Lean into God and He will help you make this shift.

As Shani began to see that Elizabeth was a narcissist, the attack seemed less personable. A narcissist will treat anyone in the same manner that gets in his or her way. Stirring up a group that will bond and come against the person is another classic maneuver. Dr. Northrup has said such a person reminds her of the wicked witch and her flying monkeys in the *Wizard of Oz*. What a great visual of a narcissist and her cohorts who do her dirty bidding!

If you've been attacked by a narcissist, please know there are support groups available. I also recommend working with a licensed therapist. An objective person who can help you grow and heal.

Step Four: Pray for guidance from God to truly see the person who hurt you through the eyes of love. Put on spiritual eyes after being hurt. This, the hardest step, is a supernatural act of God.

Only after the third step, seeing the person as wounded, can you shift to a place of compassion. Again, only with spiritual eyes can you make this leap! Pray big for God to show you how He sees this person. He will show you!

Re-scripting happens next.

With the information of what was done to you, you have the ability to rescript—to see it from a different angle. The key here is to lock down a wandering, beguiling mind with truth and love.

The fact is we are all wounded and hurting on some level. As we see each other with love and compassion, true healing occurs for all parties.

Step Five: Forgive.

You know you have forgiven when you are no longer chewing on the offense. You can see a new script, and you have shifted out of victim mode. You are truly ready to release and let go! You do not have to forget what the person or people did, but you are no longer expending energy on it. Focusing on the good and love in others allows the love to grow deeper and larger in you. That's a great win-win for all of us. Remember: love creates an environment for miracles!

As for Shani, I begged her to start a children's musical theatre program at the local shelter where I would speak and serve homeless women and children. Her family ended up moving to another state. She was able to leave in peace as she forgave, and now sees each mother in the drama group through eyes of love.

And for Elizabeth, yikes! I recently got a phone call from guess-who! "Oh, Elizabeth, I'm booked right now. No, I cannot do lunch. Thank you very much!" Wink, wink!

CHAPTER SIX

Stand Strong,
Hold Your Ground

**"The circles of women around us weave invisible
nets of love that carry us when we are weak and
sing with us when we are strong."**
Sark

It's no secret that I'm a huge animal lover. Dogs, cats, horses—
you name it, I love them all. I read a true story about a
greyhound that was left in a shed in England. Flea-infested
and skin and bones, she was brought to the local wildlife
sanctuary. It took several weeks, but eventually the staff won
over the greyhound's trust and restored her to full health. They
named her Jasmine and started looking for a foster home for
her. Before long, they noticed the effect she had on the other
animals.

When strays were brought into the sanctuary, Jasmine
would find a way to welcome them. Her warmth and affection
towards the other creatures were astounding. First thing in

the morning, she would go around to each cage and make sure everyone was alright. She would do the same with the fox and badger cubs. She would lick the rabbits and the guinea pigs, and even let the birds perch on her nose. She nurtured them in a way that took away all their stress. The other animals not only felt close to Jasmine, but also free to settle into their new environment. She made them feel safe, warm and loved. Jasmine, the previously timid, abused, and deserted one, stepped into a role for which she was born. She found her special purpose to love and nurture all—a beautiful lesson to learn from this graceful greyhound.

Hero Story

Kim Vandewater was fifty-three when she was diagnosed with breast cancer. On top of that, her mother and her best friend died, and she lost her job. Instead of pursuing another sales and marketing position, she opened a mobile pet-grooming business. Grooming rescue pets pro bono represents a significant part of her work. Her message: it's never too late and you are never too old to pursue your dreams.

Jasmine reminds me of another beautiful soul, Rainey. We met at the local shelter where I serve homeless women. I was there speaking for about three hundred ladies when I noticed her in the audience. Her gorgeous auburn hair that fell over her shoulders in silky ringlets, hazel green eyes, and striking features all stood out. She had a radiance and beauty about her. Importantly, Rainey has such a big heart to serve and love others. Her dream was to help women coming out of prostitution by launching a nonprofit.

Nevertheless, Rainey, like many other wounded ones who have no one tend to their soul, found me. Somehow, they always do. As she and I spoke, I knew immediately after that we needed to get together.

Rainey's first session was filled with tears, yet she was holding back. I knew something horrible had happened, but she was shut down and scared to share. It took a few sessions and serving at the shelter one more time for her to open up.

"That's when I met Sonia," Rainey shared, referring to how she began speaking at her church and other events to garner support for the nonprofit she envisioned. "She seemed like such a sweet, caring lady. I could hardly believe I was speaking to an audience of three hundred at a very nice church on the ritzy side of town. I was hoping for much needed resources to pour into the charity. Sonia Tindale approached me afterwards and said she wanted to help build my cause."

"I was truly flattered and excited to have a new contact and friend to help," Rainey continued. "As I got to know Sonia, she became so involved in my life. She was twenty-five years older than I and quickly became a mother figure. She helped me with my speaking events and even found a local agency that would help book me for speaking events to rally support from the community. Running a nonprofit is stressful. I had so much pressure on me and felt like I was cracking under the seams."

One of the things I loved about Rainey was the reason she wanted to help the ladies struggling with prostitution: She, too, had been set free from that lifestyle. Rainey suffered a rape at the young age of fifteen, causing her life to spin out of control on drugs and promiscuity. After marrying the man of her dreams in her twenties, she was able to get some counseling and heal the fragments of abuse. As she built her family, having three precious children, she wanted to give back and reach back to those who were lost, hurting and wounded just as she once was.

Hmmm. Her story sounded a lot like Jasmine the greyhound. I loved Rainey's big heart and still do!

"If I could turn back time, this is the moment I would," Rainey confided. "I was so stressed out with raising the kids, running the charity, speaking and ministering to women caught in prostitution, I started having some memories of my own abuse."

I explained to Rainey that memories can unfold in layers. Like the layers of an onion, each needs to be peeled back and dealt with.

"I'm sure you have healed some of those layers," I offered, "yet as stress kicks in, more layers and more memories tend to surface. Eventually," I reassured Rainey, "you get to the end of it and release it all."

I noted that if she were not finished with the work, then more issues would rise to the surface. In times of heavy stress, she wouldn't have the reserves to contain them. Like a full cup overflowing, her memories wouldn't have a hiding place. They'd rise to the top and spew out in current-day situations.

"Yes," Rainey, replied, conveying that she understood the process. "Sonia insisted that I get in counseling. She had a close friend, a pastor and counselor, who had officiated at her daughter's wedding. Sonia just insisted that I see him. She actually offered to pay for my sessions."

"The sessions with Pastor Sid started out just fine," Rainey said, "and I was opening up to him. It was strange that he would take me into an office in the back of the building that had no windows, but I trusted Sonia so much. After all, he was a friend of the family. I also trusted Pastor Sid with my heart and soul as I poured out abuse memories. I began to get closer and closer to him. He diagnosed me with post-traumatic stress disorder or PSTD, a diagnosis I had previously received."

PTSD develops in some individuals from experiencing a shocking, scary, or dangerous situation. Feeling afraid during and after a traumatic event is natural. The fight-or-flight response—a reaction in which fear triggers immediate changes within the body as a defensive or avoidance mechanism—occurs to protect a person from harm. While almost all humans experience certain reactions after some kind of trauma, most instinctively recover from the initial symptoms. Those who continue to experience problems may suffer with PTSD. A symptom of PTSD is feeling stressed or frightened even when one is not in danger.

"Pastor Sid," Rainey shared, "scheduled me for several two-hour sessions, telling me that an hour session was just not long enough. I was all on board. Eager to heal, I booked a babysitter for the kids. When I arrived for that longer session, Pastor Sid said he had a special technique which would pull out the traumatized little parts trapped within my soul so they could heal. I believe it was a form of hypnosis or something along those lines. He gave me a cup of some sort of juice to drink, stating it would keep me hydrated for the difficult session ahead."

The first two-hour session was blurry for Rainey. She could not remember clearly what was happening. Rainey remembered a hand fondling her breast and a voice telling her to rub herself and play with her private parts. Rainey's memories were in and out. Pastor Sid counted her back to consciousness, and she was grateful to be fully dressed and lying on his couch.

"Pastor Sid said, 'That was good, good work. The little abused parts came out and expressed themselves,'" Rainey remembered. "I felt a little uneasy, but when he wanted me to schedule another two-hour session for the following week, I agreed."

89

The entire week, she tried to push down the brief memory of a man's hand fondling her breast, but it consistently stayed with her. Rainey continued to feel uneasy as the next session came up. She was shaking walking into his office, and she did not know why. Rainey thought it was more abuse memories surfacing up to the top.

Rainey continued, "Again, Pastor Sid insisted on me drinking a little juice before the session to stay hydrated. 'As this is difficult work we are doing,' he would say. I remember Pastor Sid had me lay on the couch, and again he used the same technique. I was out cold until I clearly came out of the hypnotic state he'd put me in, and there I was, naked on his couch. His hands were all over me. He kept saying, 'Now, rub yourself; that's a good, good girl.' I was shocked and trapped, so I acted like I was still in a hypnotic state until he was done fondling all my body parts. I completely froze up, not knowing what to do. I acted like I was coming out of hypnosis, dressed and left. Again, Pastor Sid had assured me that I had done a great work with the little abused fragments of my soul."

Rainey screamed and cried the whole way home. "You idiot! You idiot!" she yelled. How could she be so stupid to trust this pastor? Her head was throbbing, and her mouth felt like it had when she used to do drugs: cottonmouth, as if full of cotton. Rainey was so dehydrated that she had to pull over and get water at a local gas station.

"How could I tell Dave, my husband, what had happened? And what about Sonia, my mentor; he was her family pastor. I felt sick. A huge panic came over me. I wanted to vomit and almost did. I did not know whom to tell or what to do," said Rainey.

"I got home, and Dave said, 'Are you alright?' I said, yes, I just need some rest. He thought I'd had a rough therapy session. I fell asleep sobbing into my pillow. I knew Dave would be the first I would share with, but I waited until the next day when he came home from work. It was so difficult."

If that was not bad enough, Pastor Sid called Rainey's cell phone, stating they forgot to set up another appointment. She had to remember that he did not know that she could recall what had happened. Although Rainey was unclear if that first two-hour session had involved just her abuse memories, she knew exactly what had occurred the second time. She told Pastor Sid she would have to get back to him.

Dave was burning mad with anger. Not knowing whom to call, he paced the floor back and forth for an hour. Pastor Sid was a referral for counseling through the church. Finally, Dave said he just had to confront him! Dave's call to Pastor Sid set off a ricochet of phone calls. Predators are good at what they do. Pastor Sid had been a detective in the police force before he discovered his "calling from God." He understood plausible deniability and caught on quickly that he had been busted. He called Sonia and twisted the story.

In her hypnotic state, Pastor Sid told Sonia, Rainey had ripped off her clothes and thrown herself at him. Ready with what others might accept as a logical explanation, he further said that victims with PTSD have alters in their personality, and while he and Rainey were doing the therapy work, a very strong alter of her personality had surfaced. Sonia fell for it and quickly rallied an entourage of support on the pastor's behalf.

Dave went to Pastor Sid's office and he pulled the same stunt on her husband.

"Pastor Sid said, 'Dave, your wife had a post-traumatic blow and was reliving the abuse from the past. It felt real to her, but I had nothing to do with it.' Dave told him, 'I don't believe you and I never will.' It was wonderful to have my husband's support. I don't know what I would have done without Dave at the time. We grew close and we clung to each other."

Rainey continued to tell me her story:

"Here's the second mistake I made. I had a very close relationship with my brother Eric. He had always been one of my dearest friends and a tremendous support throughout the years, especially throughout my abuse in my teen years. Why would I have thought that I could not share with him? I could always trust Eric and his caring, listening ear and heart. He was always such a great big brother. I guess, in my insecurities and outrage over the situation, I wanted to share with people who cared. I wanted my closest friends and family to be there for me. I shared everything with Eric. Ending the call, thinking he was with me and for me, I slept well that night. What more could I want? I had my husband and my brother's support. Little did I know, he called the church that night, setting off another ricochet of calls."

"Next phone call I get, I realize my brother had sided with Pastor Sid. Suddenly, I'm an unstable, adulterous liar! Oh, Victoria, it was the shock of a lifetime. My dear brother became an accuser and a betrayer."

Being a confirmed bachelor, Eric had far too much time to talk, and gossip reigned supreme. Dave and Rainey sat back and watched the enemy come through on so many calls. And, finally, the call she dreaded the most came from Sonia! If her brother wasn't the straw that broke the camel's back, Sonia hit the final nail that laid the coffin.

"She said to me, over and over, 'you are just a liar,' and then she said, 'I'll give you credit; it's not you, it's an altered personality that did it, and if you say she did not, you are a liar!'"

"Liar, liar, liar" is all that rang through Rainey's head, repeatedly. It was so ironic because all she did was tell the truth.

"Dave was determined to put the pieces together and figure out what really happened during those two, two-hour long sessions. He sat me down and said, 'Tell every last detail,'" Rainey said. "Dave and I had been married for ten years, and he had never met a strong, altered personality in me. He had seen fragmented pieces that were abused, but never a strongly aggressive part. The fragments were weepy and afraid when they would surface to the top, but I would never lose full consciousness."

Pastor Sid's story just did not add up. Dave drilled Rainey over and over until a light bulb lit up for him: the juice before the sessions.

"'Did you drink it both times?' he asked me."
"'Yes,'" I told him. 'Yes!'"
"'You were drugged!' Dave proclaimed to me. He also asked, 'Did he want you to do anything specific after the sessions?'"
"'Yes,' I answered. I told Dave that Pastor Sid had a pot of coffee brewing in his office, and he had Coca-Colas in his small refrigerator. Again, he insisted on caffeine, stating the work can make you groggy. Also, I was completely dehydrated with cottonmouth after each session."
"'That's it!' Dave shouted. 'You were drugged for these sessions.'"

As soon as he said it, Rainey knew it was exactly what happened. Dave went on to do some research on the rape drugs.

He believed Pastor Sid was giving small doses of Rohypnol in the juice. After speaking with several doctors, Dave found out that a very small amount could leave a person groggy for a short period of time. Would it be possible to be groggy for only two hours? The doctor had said, yes, absolutely, confirming Dave's suspicions.

While intended as a prescription sedative, such as for a pre-operation anesthetic or strong sleeping aid, Rohypnol, also known as roofies, has been used a date-rape drug with cases reported in the U.S., Europe, Australia. Strong doses can cause amnesia.

My heart absolutely broke in a million pieces for Rainey. She'd lost her mentor, her brother, and the support of her church all in one swing of the bat! Damn, it pissed me off! I have to say that what I learn in counseling sometimes pisses me off and this was one of those times.

Keeping my composure, I said, "First of all, Rainey, I want you to know that I believe you. I believe you are communicating the truth about Pastor Sid. I believe he drugged you and sexually abused you in his office. I also want to thank you for having the courage to share. I'm also very proud that you are still serving and blessing the prostitutes at the shelter. That takes so much courage! Do you realize how amazingly strong and resilient you are?"

Giving her a moment to take in what I'd offered, I said, "We have a lot of work to do. Is there anything else you need to share with me?"

"Yes," she said. "About three months after all this came out, I got sick. Very sick. It started with severe anemia and turned into inflammation. I guess my body could not handle all the stress."

"That's a huge amount of stress," I acknowledged, "and to lose a family member's support in addition, that's a lot of loss. Your body needs to heal from the additional trauma. I want to start by sharing 'Plato's Cave' to explain why everyone turned on you. And, by the way, Dave is my hero! Love that guy!"

That got Rainey to smile.

Allegory of the Cave

"Allegory of the Cave" is a story from Book VII from the Greek philosopher Plato's *The Republic.* The work was written in 517 BCE.

In his tale, Plato presents a cave in which prisoners are tied to some rocks. Their arms and legs are bound, and their heads are tied so that they cannot look at anything but the stone wall in front of them. Each prisoner has been there since birth; not one has ever been outside of the cave.

A fire burns behind the prison, and a raised walkway exists between the fire and the prisoners. People outside the cave use the walkway as they carry animals, plants, stone, and wood on their heads.

Imagine that you are one of the prisoners, unable to look at anything behind or to the side of you. As people passed, you'd see shadows of them with their objects on the wall before you. You'd believe that the shadows were real.

One day, a prisoner escapes the binding and leaves the cave. He is shocked at the world he discovers outside the cave. At first, he doesn't believe his eyes. As he becomes accustomed to his new surroundings, he embraces that his former view of reality was wrong. Loving the trees, the sunshine, the animals, and other individuals, he sees that his former life was useless. The escaped prisoner decides to return to the cave to inform the others. Not only do they believe he is lying, but they also threaten to kill him if he tries to set them free! The truth was too scary for the prisoners, set in their ways.

When someone shines the light and brings truth, some groups remain closed to seeing the truth!

After sharing the story, I told Rainey some people might be threatened by the truth. They do not want to see it. All you can do is work on yourself. If people want to remain in their caves and see only shadows, then you must honor them and their journey. As you heal, forgive and release them, you find yourself in a stronger place. At that point, you can even turn back and say thank you for the lessons learned. It is possible for you to heal and grow even if others stay stuck in their shadowy caves. As you continue to grow and even look deeper, you come to know that their shadows are really a reflection of our own shadows as well.

"Let me explain more deeply," I offered. "Sonia, your mentor, could never see that Pastor Sid was a predator. For her to admit this would mean a predator had officiated at her daughter's wedding and been a friend of the family for years. This was way too scary for her to admit. How could she justify that? Sometimes the truth hurts deeply.

"Your brother chose to hang out in the shadows," I continued. "He could not see the truth due to a lack of seeing your success. Many families have members who are stuck in old roles."

As Rainey grew, became healed, and birthed a nonprofit, her brother had a difficult time letting go of her old role as the family prostitute. He chose not to see the new Rainey. That saddened me the most. I know how much this wound hurts, especially since he was once supportive.

To comfort Rainey, I said, "We will do some deep, inner-healing work on this. You can learn to rescript this and see him in his wounded self. That's exactly what we will do. We will rescript Eric and eventually see him through the eyes of compassion."

Rainey shared that the church continued to keep Pastor Sid as a referral for others to receive counseling. Several times when Rainey went for group prayer, a female pastor at the church would see her and say, "If you have lied or if you are a liar, you need to repent." In response, Rainey and Dave made the healthy decision to move on to another church. It's frightening to think that a church would be so interested in protecting their pastor's reputation that they were willing to allow others to be abused.

I'm delighted to see movements like Me Too coming to the forefront, so ladies can be heard. It's time to speak up and speak out. If you have been abused, find a safe person with whom you can share. Let's all work to provide a safe environment to heal and grow. As in Rainey's case, many family members will not only be unsupportive, but also turn on the victim. Cheers for her husband Dave, who could see the truth. I'm proud of you Rainey, so, so proud of you for your courage to get this healed!

Saltwater Tip: Two Healing Exercises

Healing Exercise #1: Sword and Torch

My friend Brenda from Alabama and I love to look up the meanings of names. The Scottish origin of *Brenda* comes from the Norse words for *sword* and *torch*. The name spread from the Shetland Isles of Scotland to other parts of the English-speaking world after the character Brenda appeared as a heroine in Sir Walter Scott's 1822 novel, *The Pirate*. Fittingly, Brenda shared an inner healing exercise with me that involves a sword and a torch. We've used it with many ladies who have been abused.

The premise is that we have soul ties that form when we have sex with others. Soul ties stick. Even though we can pray over the circumstances, the ties and wounds can be tough to break. Like a stain on a shirt that requires some scrubbing with detergent before tossing it in the wash, removing this kind of stain on the soul needs some deep work.

Close your eyes. Taking a deep breath, breathe in and breathe out three times. Breathe in through the nostrils and out through the mouth.

Coaching Rainey through this exercise, I said, "I want you to visualize Pastor Sid. Get a visual of him and be still. What are you experiencing in your body? Do you sense that he is connected to you? Are you feeling any sensations on your chest, back, or stomach?"

Rainey said, "Yes, I'm feeling pressure in my stomach and on my back."

"Continue to feel this," I said, "and tell me what you see."

"I feel bound . . . constricted," Rainey revealed, "like a snake has wrapped itself around me, squeezing me. And I can't breathe. I can't move. It's very restrictive and I can't move my arms. I'm trapped."

"Okay," I said, "trust this image and I want you to prepare to release yourself. Can you slide one hand through and have it break free? Visualize doing this."

"Yes," Rainey said, "I have one hand free."

"This snake," I explained, "is a visual of a trapped and bound soul. It's causing a huge imbalance. Now visualize a sword in your hand. You are going to break free. Now lower the sword and swiftly cut the snake."

Rainey literally lifted her hand as I instructed and held a visualization of a sword, which cut through the snake.

"It might take several times," I let her know. Sh repeated the motions and I said, "Okay, good. Now watch it fall to the ground and disappear. Now see Pastor Sid standing before you. He has no power over you. Now release him."

Rainey courageously said aloud, "I honor you and bless you, Pastor Sid. I release you in love. I see you in light." Tears streamed down her cheeks.

"Now repeat after me," I said. "Any negative energy I have picked up from Pastor Sid, I command it to go back to him. Any positive energy you have gleaned from me, I command my positive energy back to me. I bless, honor, love and release you, Pastor Sid!"

Rainey repeated the words.

"Now," I instructed, "light a torch, walk around in a circle, and surround yourself with the light of the torch. This is your safety zone, free from abuse and memories. Now, as you release Pastor Sid, see him in light."

Why did Rainey need to see Pastor Sid in the light?

"Anyone who claims to be in the light but hates a brother or sister is still in the darkness. Anyone who loves their brother and sister lives in the light, and there is nothing in them to make them stumble. But anyone who hates a brother or sister is in the darkness and walks around in the darkness. They do not know where they are going, because the darkness has blinded them." 1 John: 8-11

When you release the one who wronged you in his or her light, you experience the release break into freedom. This step always puts a smile on my face.

Some have seen cords, tight ropes, Slinkys—you name it—to bind them. The sword cuts any material, and you are free to release your tie to the person. You cut the soul tie loose and encircle yourself with light and love. While encircling yourself, you release and encircle the abuser with light and love. It's a high calling, and love is the best teacher.

I encourage ladies to journal after the experience. By writing, they always see more. Also, after completing this step, their capacity to love and grow expands in a deeper way.

Rainey was not quite ready for Healing Exercise #2, so she tapped to prepare herself to release the abuse and emotional pain on a cellular level. For a full explanation of tapping, please see Chapter 5.

"Okay," I said, preparing Rainey for the tapping exercise, "I want you to close your eyes. Take a deep breath in and hold it, and let it go. Just breathe comfortably with your eyes closed—feeling what goes on inside, noticing what you feel physically, noticing what you feel emotionally—and say, 'I am willing to heal the past.' Now, just take a moment and let that rattle around inside and notice what you feel. Notice on a scale of zero to ten how true that feels. Part of you might want to say it's a ten, and if it were truly a ten, it would already be done, or at least on the way. Don't judge yourself if the number is low; just allow yourself to recognize that wow, I love myself so much that I'm really holding on to this. Just allow yourself to know which thoughts, beliefs, and memories might be there, as to why you might not be fully willing. Just allow yourself to be at peace with that as much as possible and open your eyes."

From that point, I led Rainey to tap to release the hurt and wounds on a cellular level. The following indicates what to tap while speaking the affirmation:

Side of the Hand

Even though part of me resists healing, I choose to love and accept myself anyway.

Even though part of me resists healing, I choose to love and honor myself anyway.

Even though part of me resists healing, part of me says I I'm going to hang on to this hurt and I love and appreciate that part of me.

Even though I sometimes resist healing, I choose to deeply and completely love, honor, and accept myself, and maybe anyone else who has taught me to be so resistant.

Eyebrow
All this resistance to healing
Side of Eye
All this resistance to healing
Under Eye
All this fear of healing
Under Nose
All this fear that if I let some of this go
Under Mouth
I am going to be hurt.
Collarbone
I have been hurt in the past.
Under Arm
And part of me is convinced
Top of Head
That the only thing that keeps me safe now
Eyebrow
Is holding on to these memories

Side of Eye
Holding on to this pain
Under Eye
Oh sure, it causes a lot of misery too,
Under Nose
Blocks me from all kinds of opportunities.
Under Mouth
It may be robbing me of health, wealth, and happiness.
Collarbone
But I love and appreciate that part of me
Under Arm
That has become convinced
Top of Head
That I'm safer this way.
Eyebrow
And I'm allowing myself to relax.

Side of Eye
And really look at what's
necessary.
Under Eye
What do I really need to
hang on to?
Under Nose
What can I let go?
Under Mouth
And I choose to have more
faith in myself.
Collarbone
I choose to be willing
to heal.
Under Arm
I choose to know that I can
handle healing.
Top of Head
I can handle the freedom
that comes with that.
Eyebrow
I can handle this.

Side of Eye
I have handled everything
else that's happened in
my life.
Under Eye
Maybe not always as
gracefully as I would have
liked.
Under Nose
But I'm still here.
Under Mouth
Which means I have
handled it.
Collarbone
I can handle healing.
Under Arm
I am allowing myself to be
willing to heal,
Top of Head
In body, mind, and spirit.

"Now," I coached Rainey. "Take a deep breath. Close your eyes again, and again feeling inside, particularly if there was some sensation you were aware of before, on a scale of zero to ten, how willing do you feel now to allow yourself to heal and move forward? Hopefully that number has gone way up, and it may be that because tapping is like peeling layers of the onion, through the tapping you have allowed yourself to become more aware of why you might still be holding on to things and just allow yourself to recognize that and say, okay, that's where I am going to start tapping."

Rainey's number went way up; she truly was ready for healing.

I want to thank Brad Yates and The Tapping Summit for this Tapping Script. You can find information about Brad Yates and the Magnificent Tappers, along with other resources, in the back of this book.

After tapping, Rainey and I proceeded to the next healing exercise. Our sessions were done on different days, so please pace yourself on your healing journey. Always, check with a Licensed Professional Therapist when dealing with issues of abuse or traumatic experiences.

Healing Exercise #2: Allowing Compassion

After the first exercise and tapping, Rainey was ready for the second healing exercise.

Rainey had forgiven Pastor Sid and even Sonia, but the harder person to forgive was her brother. To allow compassion, she had to shift her thinking. That shift took time and work.

I encouraged Rainey to list what she liked about her brother—a challenge because a loving friend and brother had morphed into a religious, pompous judger. Pausing to prevent judging, we worked through the shock of his actions and reached the realization that he was just acting out of his own wounded emotions. That was a big shift for Rainey.

In dysfunctional families, siblings take on different roles. Rainey acted out as a black sheep of the family after abuse. Her brother Eric became the parent of the family, an unnatural role for a child, in an out-of-control situation. When he heard what happened with Pastor Sid, he felt out of control, so he called the church to grab control. It was never his place to make that phone call, and that leads to another problem with dysfunction: boundaries. Eric broke boundaries and lost his loyalty to his sister.

Grieving the loss of her brother and the deep friendship they had, Rainey was able to move on. She started re-scripting by looking back on the supportive brother she once knew. Before long, memories of supportive days, when her brother was loving, flooded back. Remembering caused a shift in Rainey: moving off the script of "religious prick" and "asshole" to times when she remembered him as a loving, caring brother and friend.

Oh, the adjectives come out when we do this amazing work! I truly want it all to come out, and then the shift to compassion is amazing.

Rainey could see her brother in his shadows and embrace him—wounds and all. Truly, he was just a little kid trying to control out-of-control "things" as he was growing up. The scare with Rainey and Pastor Sid drove him back to the wounded little kid. As Rainey could see this, she moved into forgiveness. She repeated after me, "I love you in your shadows, and I love you in your light, and I can see you through the eyes of love and compassion." What a shift!

Practicing re-scripting and seeing with compassion releases you from the bondage of judgement.

Rainey skipped down my driveway to her car that day. I saw a light in her eyes spark back up as she released judgement of her brother. As Rainey re-scripted the events, she remembered her caring brother yet saw him in his shadows of judgement and hurt as well. Now she prays for him to heal and grow as well. Beautiful work!

Seeing the person who hurt you through the eyes of God is a supernatural happening.

Rainey went on to rock it with a powerful and successful nonprofit! As she did her healing work, God blessed her on all fronts with her marriage, her children, and her nonprofit all thriving!

Can we all say, God is good!

Just like Jasmine the beautiful greyhound, Rainey has continued in her work at the shelter, loving and caring for those who are finding their way to healing, too. Rainey is a bright light in the community, sharing love and healing to all. Instead of shutting down in resentment and bitterness, she did the hard work to heal, and God met her in the midst of it. What a beautiful journey!

I love you, precious Rainey!

CHAPTER SEVEN

This is What Friends are For!

Bad Hair Day! Ain't nobody got time for that!

"Girls, I'm home!" Terri called.

Terri's two daughters, Katie, age twelve, and Lauren, age ten, looked up from their show on Nickelodeon.

"Hey, I was talking to Victoria," Terri said, "and she encouraged me to highlight my hair. I'm going to do it. Yes, I'm going to do it!"

The girls jumped up off the couch. "Yes, Mom! We want to help you do it!"

"I don't know," Terri said, suddenly hesitant. "This could be complicated. Well, I did buy this hair dye at the store. Yeah, maybe you two should help me."

After reading the directions and washing her hair, she donned plastic gloves and one of her husband Bubba's old work shirts. Following the directions, they mixed the hair dye with the developer (the latter of which enables the dye to penetrate). Using the correct proportions would be essential. Even with the girls' enthusiasm, Terri had made sure they had applied the highlights correctly by carefully wrapping the right amount of hair and dye in each section of foil. They were all so pleased that it looked as if a professional had done the job. The only question was how long to wait before rinsing. The box had been ripped just a bit where the time was printed. It appeared to read three hours.

"Mom, that seems like a long time," said Katie.

Thinking her sister would know, Terri tried phoning her, but she didn't answer.

"Let's just go with three hours," she said.

To pass the time, they ordered pizza for dinner and watched a movie. Finally, the buzzer signaled that she could remove the foil wraps and wash her hair. As Terri emerged from the shower with a towel wrapped around her, Lauren, the first to see her mom's hair, held her breath. Terri, busy with the blow-dryer, didn't react at first. After a few moments, however, she glanced in the mirror.

"It's green! It's green!" Terri screamed.

Hearing the ruckus, Bubba ran in to find out what was wrong.

"Lordy, Lordy, Terri! You've ruined your hair! What will you do? Cut it all off?"
"Get out!" Terri screamed. "Get out, Bubba!"

The girls didn't know whether to laugh or cry, were mostly laughing.

That same evening, close to ten o'clock, my cell rang.

Jeff looked at it and said, "Do you ladies ever quit talking?"

I smiled and said, "No!" Seeing Terri's name, I cheerfully said, "Hi, Terri."

Immediately, she began shouting, "I ruined my hair! I ruined my hair!"

"What? Calm down," I interjected, striving to remain calm. "What happened?"

"Well, I took you up on your suggestion to do highlights, but I guess I thought I'd save money by doing it myself," she began. "And the girls helped me!"

"What? You and the girls did your highlights?" I asked. "I did not know you did hair."

That was definitely not the right thing to say.

"I don't!" Terri was almost screaming at me.

"Okay, okay," I responded. "Calm down."

"You don't understand," she continued. "It's green!"

"How green?" I bravely asked.

"Very green and an ugly green!" she barked.

Somehow, this was all my fault, so I'd better offer a good solution.

"Okay," Terri, "I know just the person to call: Adrienne. She has some fancy hairdresser who comes to her home. He's from Buckhead," I added, referring to an area of Atlanta that draws a wealthy clientele. "I'll call her first thing in the morning."

Still exasperated, Terri wondered what she was supposed to do in the meantime.

"My advice," I said, "is to wear a hat in the morning carpool line."

Suggesting that Bubba probably had a baseball cap she could borrow seemed to calm her down at last, and she thanked me between sniffles.

I couldn't help but laugh when I got off the phone.

"What was that all about?" Jeff asked.

"No big deal," I filled him in. "Terri dyed her hair green."

"What! You ladies are something else," Jeff chuckled, as he went upstairs. "Never dull; never, ever dull!"

Jeff left early the next morning with a full day on his plate. After I took care of my doggies, Adrienne was at the top of my list to call. When I picked up my phone, I found I'd already received a text from Terri, eager to know if I had called Adrienne. Quickly, I got in touch Adrienne and shared the story of Terri's green hair.

"We need your hairdresser," I explained.

Adrienne not only agreed to contact Frederic (pronounced Fre•dé•ric), but also graciously offered to pay his fee, which Terri could not afford.

"That's what friends are for!" Adrienne pronounced.

Serving an elite clientele, Frederic had made a big name for himself in New York City. His former partner had passed away, leaving him quite wealthy. Moving to Midtown in the heart of downtown Atlanta with Marlo, his new partner, Frederic not only catered to the rich and famous, but he also lived among them. His home was near Elton John's place! Adrienne had met Frederic and Marlo at a dinner party and immediately fell in love with them. Experts in private spa parties, hair, nails, facials, and massage, they make you feel like a queen for a day. But have your wallet ready!

I was out walking my Aussies a little later when Adrienne called back to say that she had hired them for a spa day at her home on Saturday.

"Clear your schedule and call Terri now," she said. "They had a big cancellation, and this is unheard of!"

Hormone Level Test

I had been hoping Adrienne could arrange a hairdo fix for Terri, who had been struggling with some perimenopausal issues. Such struggles can make relatively small matters seem huge. Admittedly, green hair would be upsetting, but it wasn't the end of the world.

Smile!

As Terri and I had discussed, you may need to have your levels of estrogen, progesterone, DHEA, testosterone, and other hormones tested. At the same time, pay attention to how you feel, which can be a far more accurate way to assess hormone balance than simply relying on a lab test. Combining lab results with how you feel allows you and your doctor to customize a treatment plan that is right for you. When the need arises to supplement, many doctors recommend that you start with the lowest dose possible and see how you do.

Also, as discussed in Chapter 3, change your diet to a low-sugar, organic-food approach. Add a natural herbal remedy such as Pueraria mirifica, maca, black cohosh, ground golden flaxseed, or chasteberry. If that strategy doesn't work, then try the bioidenticals.

Saltwater Tip: Add a natural herbal remedy, such as Pueraria mirifica, maca, black cohosh, ground golden flaxseed, or chasteberry.

The Difference Between Bioidentical Hormones and Synthetic Hormones

As the term bioidentical implies, bioidentical hormones are blended to be an exact match in molecular structure to a woman's body. In contrast, non-bioidentical (synthetic) estrogen, such as the estrogen in a drug like Premarin, is bioidentical only if you're a horse. Yes, the estrogen in Premarin is made from the urine of pregnant horses.

Progestin, a synthetic form of progesterone, is derived from bioidentical progesterone. A bioidentical hormone is naturally occurring, so it cannot be patented. Therefore, to make progesterone marketable, the compound was altered to make Progestin, which is not native to the female human body.

For about two decades, doctors primarily recommended Premarin (the synthetic estrogen) and Prempro (a synthetic form of progesterone). The protocol changed in 2002, when the Women's Health Initiative Studies found that supplementing with synthetics—estrogen or progesterone—increased the risk of breast cancer, heart attack, stroke, and blood clots. Comparisons included studies with women given placebos.

My advice is to choose a natural herbal remedy. If herbals don't work, try bioidentical hormones.

My sister died of cancer, so I refuse to take Premarin or Prempro. Again, I'm not a doctor, and I would not suggest that you take my advice over what your medical professional recommends. Nevertheless, don't let a doctor intimidate you into thinking you cannot get a second or third or fourth opinion. Consult with multiple doctors and educate yourself regarding your options—pros and cons—before trying hormones.

Green Hair Gone

Continuing my walk with a skip and a jump, I was about to call Terri, but realized I needed to ask Adrienne how much getting the royal treatment would cost me.

I called her back and she said, "Oh, darlin', no worries! It's all on me this time." I asked if she were certain, and she said, "Yes, I insist!"

I hung up wondering what was going on with Adrienne. She was a lovely person, but not really one to treat, even though she was financially well off. Her husband had died unexpectedly five years before, leaving her as the controlling shareholder of a thriving business. We had all been heartbroken and shocked by his death Seemingly in excellent shape, he had gone out jogging one morning, grabbed his chest during a massive heart attack, and passed away later at the hospital. We all admired Adrienne's strength.

When I called Terri, she said, "Well, it's about time."
I didn't let her frustration get to me. Instead, I asked her to sit down before announcing Adrienne's news: "Adrienne got Frederic and Marlo for Saturday! Clear the deck—we have a spa day at St. Ives."

St. Ives is one of North Atlanta's gated country-club communities. Terri right away said she couldn't afford it, so I took great pleasure in relaying that Adrienne would be treating us. How great to hear glee in her voice rather than gloom!
When Saturday morning arrived with a gorgeous sunrise, I decided to make the most of the experience by borrowing Jeff's Mini Cooper and driving to Adrienne's with the top down. Feeling the breeze and seventy-degree temperature, I was thinking that life, indeed, was good.

Terri and I showed up at the same time. Emerging from the car, I yelled, "Take the hat off, Terri. Let me see it!"

Terri yanked off the Atlanta Braves Baseball cap she'd borrowed from Bubba, and I screamed and started laughing hysterically.

She initially laughed, but then started crying. I hugged her, saying, "It will be alright, honey. Let's go in." I couldn't help myself, however, by adding, "I just have to say, Terri, that is the ugliest green I've ever seen."

She wasn't happy, so I changed the subject as we took the walkway to Adrienne's front door, mentioning the multimillion-dollar price listed for a mansion a few houses away. Terri shook her head in disbelief.

"We are hobnobbing with the rich and famous!" I exclaimed.

At last, Terri cracked a smile.
Frederic himself greeted us at the door.

"Hello," he said with flourish, "I'm Fre•dé•ric, and you two ladies must be Victoria and Terri! Marlo and I have been here for an hour getting ready for you ladies. Marlo is an excellent cook, and he has prepared a wonderful breakfast for you of fruits, gluten-free Eggs Benedict, and Bloody Marys to kick off the morning. And don't say no! You are here to indulge. You can pay for it tomorrow, but today you play."

We entered the foyer, featuring a grand circular staircase, and then stepped into a sunken living room with rounded walls. Curved windows with beautiful stained glass flanked a stone fireplace. I was afraid to touch anything. The mansion was not only spectacular, but also immaculate, and Adrienne's furnishings all wore light colors. We continued to follow Frederic, who guided us to the backyard with a stone patio and infinity pool. A wooded land preserve bordered the property, creating a secluded retreat. Spotting some deer, I thought how much my dogs would love playing here.

Greeting us, Adrienne warmly expressed how happy she was to have us join her. Marlo, the perfectly handsome image of a Greek god, approached us with a tray of Bloody Marys.

"Ladies help yourself!" he declared. "We have plenty."

Assuring us that they were there to pamper us, Marlo and Frederic began to do just that. After sharing a good laugh over Terri's do-it-yourself salon experience, this time with Terri acknowledging the humor in it, we savored our breakfast and sipped our drinks. Soon, Frederic whisked Terri away to restore her hair, and Adrienne and I rotated between massages and saunas.

With my face slathered in therapeutic mud and my eyelids covered with freshly sliced cucumbers, I was peacefully alone in a dimly lit sanctuary of warmth and the scent of lavender. Soft music blended with sounds of the ocean, and Marlo had set me up so that I could sip my cocktail through a straw. Actually, I had been zipped into a portable sauna, like a mini tent, inside a private room by the pool. For the moment, I was in heaven. Letting all the cares of the day and my life melt away, I could feel the stress leaving my body. I took another sip of my Bloody Mary and noticed the ice had melted in the drink. Yes, it was getting warmer, but the heat felt good.

Breathing in and out, mediating, and trying to clear my mind, I thought to myself, this is getting really hot. This is almost uncomfortably hot. I took another sip of my decidedly warm cocktail, and all of sudden, a big hot flash encompassed my body. Oh, no! I had forgotten that the alcohol contained sugar, a cause of hot flashes—at least, for me it did. Oh, yeah, I also remembered, I don't even drink. What was I thinking? I was hot flashing to the point of unbearable discomfort.

"Hey, Marlo!" I screamed. "It's time for me to get out! Marlo!"

He didn't respond. Darn! No one can hear me. Oh, okay, I thought, there's a zipper on the inside. However, the darn cucumbers were stuck to my eyelids, so I couldn't see a thing. Rubbing with my hand to knock off a cucumber was impossible. Where is that zipper? I felt around with my hand, but no zipper. I was stuck holding this bloody Bloody Mary, which was as hot as the devil, and my arm had grown tired of holding it up. My only escape was to hop to freedom—in other words, exit the room while still zipped inside the sauna. Bad idea or not, I had to get out of that hot box! Hot flashes were rearing their ugly head.

Upon taking a couple of hops to the door, I could see that my sauna was hooked up to something by a long extension cord. Who knew where it was plugged in! No matter, I hopped and hopped. Oops! I spilled my drink a little! Sorry, Adrienne. Yikes, Adrienne will kill me, I was thinking, but I made it to the door. With the Bloody Mary in one hand, I leaned over to turn the doorknob with the other. The door, which opened inward, did not move. My sauna was blocking the door, so I had to hop backwards. As I did, I fell backwards. Everything went black.

The next thing I saw were Adrienne and Marlo's fuzzy faces coming into focus. We all started laughing!

"Oh, my gosh" I announced. "I was hot flashing in the sauna, and I thought I was dying."

"Okay," Adrienne chuckled, "you owe me for the carpet stains."

Saltwater Tip: Enjoy the pleasures of life but remember to treat your body well.

We all wrapped up the day with our hair and nails. Terri's hair was gorgeous—back to her golden blonde!

After we said our goodbyes to Frederic and Marlo, Adrienne asked Terri and me to sit down with her in her living room. We thanked her again for the fabulous day, and Adrienne let us know that she wanted us to have the special memory of being together.

"You guys have become so important to me over the last few years," she said. "After my husband's death, you have been among just a few who have stuck by me. I love you both dearly. I shudder to think what I'd do without you two."

Terri and I could tell the conversation was turning serious.

"I don't know what I'm facing," she continued, "but my gynecologist has found a lump in my right breast."

Terri let out a gasp. "Oh Adrienne," I said, "I am so sorry.

"The biopsy came back as Stage 2 cancer," she revealed. We were all silent. "This means the breast cancer is growing, but it is contained. There is the possibility that some cells have extended to the lymph nodes. They are preparing to do a mastectomy, which will tell more—if it's in the lymph nodes or not."

The three of us hugged and cried. For the moment, I was speechless.

When I found my voice, I said, "Let us know when, and we will be with you. You know that."

Adrienne wiped tears from her eyes and shook her head. "I'm so glad we all had this day together," she said. "This is what I wanted the most."

We all hugged. Instead of getting on my phone, I immersed myself in silence all the way home. The sun was setting as I drove into my subdivision.

CHAPTER EIGHT

Is It Hot? Oh, Yeah — Sizzling Hot!

**"You are going to get through all the hardships
and pain, but they are necessary to make
you stronger and wise."
Lynda Weinmann**

"Who wants some pie?" asked Kim, a beautiful, tall, buxom blonde.

She was holding a big apple pie with forty candles in celebration of her husband Tony's birthday. As she leaned over and set the dessert in the middle of a large picnic table, the four men sitting around the table exchanged smirks with one another and winked.

"We do," they replied in unison.

Kim, fully aware that her recent boob job was obvious, winked back at the men and said, "You bad boys."

Jolinda, meanwhile, kicked her husband under the table, causing him to shout, "Ouch!" Tony, ignoring the outburst, leaned over to blow out his candles.

Having known one another most of their lives, the four men, with their wives, would get together several times a year for what they called the Alpharetta Dinner Club. Two guys had played football in high school, and they all became buddies in college. Certainly, they recognized the rarity of a close friendship like theirs to last, but the fact that they led similar lives made it easier. All men were married with families, and they were successful in their careers.

Jolinda, married to Shannon Thomas, had worked with me years before during my corporate sales days. We managed to stay in touch, seeing each other three to four times a year, and talking over the phone often. My husband and I were always invited to her annual New Year's Day dinner party, and that's where we met the group. Jeff and I were welcomed to the Alpharetta Dinner Club, so we would pop into their restaurant gatherings and parties as our schedule allowed. Jolinda and I maintained a strong friendship through the years. Although Jeff and I were not as connected with the others, we stayed in touch with them through their New Years' parties and other get togethers, which gave us a window into their lives.

The women of the group—Jolinda, Kim, Carol and Luna—all had their children close together in age, which fostered their bonds. The men—Tony, Shannon, Dick and John—would hang out as they had in college, only they had their official "man cave" in their respective homes to watch football, drink beer, cut up, and rib each other.

Drinking was typically part of the friends' celebrations. A special occasion like Tony's fortieth birthday called for plenty of Jell-O shooters and spiked watermelon. Tony and Kim owned a beautiful boathouse with a deck on top that overlooked Lake Lanier, and we were all out on the pier. The party was going strong when Jolinda and her husband Shannon decided to leave. Kim had put Jolinda's purse somewhere for safekeeping, so Jolinda went looking through several of the bedrooms. That's when she walked in on Kim and Dick. Although Dick and Luna had three children and he claimed to be happily married, we'd heard rumors that he ran around on her.

"I opened the bedroom door, searching for my purse," Jolinda confided to me years later over lunch. "I did not think much about it then, but there was an awkward silence for a moment when I walked in on Kim and Dick in the bedroom. I assumed they were looking for Luna's purse. I thanked Kim for the lovely party and gathered my purse. We said our goodbyes. I never gave it another thought, even though now, looking back, there was that awkward silence."

Kim had always been super flirty with the men, but we all still loved her and would just think, well, that's just Kim. We continued to meet for dinner and at parties. No one would have suspected an affair.

It all came out ten years later, when John, Tony's buddy since high school, was celebrating his fiftieth birthday. His wife Carol surprised him with a big party, and she was the one who walked in on Kim and Dick that evening. Seemingly eager to get off by themselves, the illicit couple were in the garage when Carol flipped on the lights. They never would have been caught had the party not run out of ice, prompting Carol to make a quick trip to the store. Both had their pants down in the front seat of her Suburban.

"Well, I guess you two should get dressed," Carol stammered in shock.

A stay-at-home, salt-of-the-earth mom who homeschooled her kids, she would be more stunned than any of the ladies in the group by such behavior. At that point, Carol ran out of the garage and started crying. Attempting to hold herself together until the party was over, she touched up her make-up and returned to the festivities. John, however, knew something was wrong.

"Tell me what's going on, Carol," he said. "The party was awesome. We had such a great turnout."

She couldn't tell John what she'd seen, so Carol simply said that she wanted to rest. John let it go, unaware that his wife would spend the night crying into her pillow.

The next morning at breakfast, John pried the truth out of her. He was livid. To avoid upsetting Carol by making a phone call she'd overhear, he drove to Dick's home to confront him in person. Seeing that Luna and kids were not there, John barged in without knocking.

"Stop right there, John!" Dick said, throwing up his arms.

John, a Lieutenant Colonel who had faced far more formidable threats, charged at Dick with fire in his eyes.

"Dick, you've never been anything more than a life support system for a penis," he accused. "All you think about is women, sports, and airplanes." Indeed, Dick was a pilot. "I've taken up for you all these years. I've always been the one who covered for you. But this tops it. We are grownups. We are not in college! My wife's Suburban—come on, man! Don't you see that this doesn't just affect you? This affects all of us: your family, your children, your friends . . . the community!"

"Yeah, yeah, I've let everybody down," Dick said. He was aloof, not repentant.

John, having reached his breaking point, grabbed Dick and slammed him into the wall. "Don't you get it, man? We are no longer in college!"

Dick shoved back and swung at John, landing a right hook to his jaw. John stumbled backwards and righted himself.

Putting his hand up to his jaw, he said, "You idiot! After all these years, you still just don't you get it We are fifty, man! We are fifty years old! Grow up! You are going to lose Luna and the kids, and you will be alone. This will not last with Kim. This is more of your bullshit. You are going to lose everything and everyone, and you will be alone. No friendships or roots. Kids who hate you and an ex-wife. And guess what? A girlfriend who will leave you, too!"

The news broke to everyone. As John had predicted, Kim had no intention of staying with Dick. She loved the excitement of an affair and sneaking around, but she never wanted to be with the playboy pilot permanently. Luna divorced Dick. Likewise, Tony, being too humiliated to face his close friends and saying he could no longer stay, divorced Kim.

From that point on, the dinner group ran on dysfunction: making fun of Dick and his crude jokes, and snidely remarking about Kim's boobs and outfits. In truth, all of us, men and women, were hurt deeply. The last time we all met, Pete, one of the fringe members of the group, had some final words for Tony that summed up the situation. He and Tony were on the deck outside, and Pete, a doctor, was ragging Tony for vaping.

In defense, Tony said, "Guys our age vape to feel young, and young guys vape to look old." Looking down, he added, "Things will never be the same."

"That's too bad," Pete said. "This dinner club was one of the more exciting events I had to look forward to, socially. You know, Tony, bad decisions have consequences, and love has consequences. We are all connected. We are all affected by love, and love trumps all. Keep searching. There's someone out there for you who will love and respect you."

Luna moved back to her hometown in Illinois with the kids. Kim floundered like a lost puppy after Tony left her. I ran into her a couple of times, once when we were leaving a restaurant and she was arriving with a new boyfriend. She seemed to be getting a buzz on, and catching our glance, came over to say hello. We hugged.

She was quick to say, "I'm doing great, really. Business is good, and the kids and I are great."

Seeing the deep hurt in her eyes, I hugged her as tightly as I could and said, "Please, please stay in touch."

She walked off, glancing back. The pain showed.

As the friend group started unraveling, Jolinda would call me. I would try to give advice, but the circumstances finally became too much for her to handle. Meanwhile, Carol, Kim and Jolinda were all going through menopause.

After the chips had fallen, about a year after the ordeal went down, Kim finally called me for counseling. I was so glad she had the courage, especially since I had been loosely connected to the friend group through Jolinda. When she arrived at my home, however, she entered my foyer a bit uptight. I could tell she was not sure whether she could trust me or not.

"Kim, I'm so glad you made this step," I warmly greeted her.

She shook her head as if to say, I'm not sure about talking to you but I've got nothing to lose at this point. Two marriages gone bust, two broken families, hurt children, and hurt friends.

"You have to start someplace," I replied to her unspoken words.

She followed me to my upper room, and I offered her the couch or the floor with pillows. She sat on the couch.

"Kim, can you share with me a little about your background?"

"I was raised in an upper-middle class home," Kim began. Her voice was soft, and her tone was a bit untrusting, but she continued. "My father traveled and worked all the time. I have two sisters. I'm the middle child. Somehow, being in the middle, I felt left out or mixed into the pack most of the time. Mother was busy with her career and my father worked long days, often into the night. Many nights, we would not see him. In middle school, I longed for attention. I started getting attention from boys and I really liked it. I guess, from fifth grade on, I started gleaning my attention fix from boys. I became totally boy crazy. Everything I did from middle school on was to glean male attention. From batting my eyes, to wearing low-cut tops, to faking needing help with homework, I did it for attention. I started making out with guys under the staircase in middle school—sixth or seventh grade."

I asked what male attention meant to her. Kim hesitated before answering. She admitted that if she was getting that attention, it felt like "love." From eighth grade on, Kim always had a boyfriend. It became a crutch for her. Flirting with others was her "just in case" plan. She was a cheerleader in high school and was pegged as the "loose" girl because of her willingness to have sex. For Kim, high school was about partying and dating athletes. At eighteen, she was pregnant and didn't know who the father was. She didn't have time for a baby. Planning for college, she earned money by working at a department store and went alone to get her abortion. It was a lonely time, but Kim healed and went on to college. It was there she met Tony and her wider group of friends.

"Tony and I were a great couple," Kim said as the tears started streaking down her cheeks. "We just seemed to belong together."

"Kim, it will be alright," I said. "We are going to bring healing to this situation. You will see. God has a way. He moves mysteriously at times, yet healing will come to all parties who want it."

I suspected that Kim was not telling me everything. I highly suspected sexual abuse. Of course, she would have to tell me if it were true. I absolutely said nothing of my hunch.

When Kim came back to me for additional sessions, we looked at her promiscuous behavior, but not in a judging way. I was giving her insight as to what it meant for her. I wanted her to love, honor, and respect herself. I longed for her to know how very special she was. After only a few sessions, Kim burst into tears, confessing she had been sexually abused by a neighbor when she was in middle school.

My hunch had been correct. I was so grieved for her yet knew that healing would come as we looked at the difficult truths. She would face her past and get through it. As soon as she confessed, her sexual abuse memories spilled out. Kim was ready. Abuse memories and their related emotions freeze like ice cubes for self-protection. Fear as well as anger and rage commonly come out during the thawing process. Giving her a place to direct her emotions, I offered Kim an empty chair and then stepped outside with my doggies to give her all the freedom she needed. She instantly let go, screaming, hollering and saying everything she'd wanted to express back in middle school but could not.

To release anger and rage, and reach the other side, you must go back and feel all of it.

When I returned to Kim, she was finished and sobbing. The hard work, which was not over, would lead to deep healing. In the sessions to follow, we'd have to replace her outrage with good. Kim's initial effort had been a great start.

Next, she needed to love herself as she began to nurture her inner child who had been abused and neglected. To begin, I instructed Kim close her eyes and repeat the following:

I'm sending love to my inner child.

I'm sending love to my inner child, and I chose to love and honor myself.

I'm giving love to my inner child.

I recognize that child has been through some stuff. I did not know how to really take care of myself and heal.

I am sending love to my inner child and I deeply and completely love, honor and accept all of me.

I'm fully loving my inner child, giving my child a loving hug and allow the child to heal.

I'm letting my inner child know we are deserving of love, feeling all the love and moving forward with lots of love.

"Now," I said, "give yourself a big hug!"

When Kim was ready to leave that day, I instructed her to pray, asking God to show her how special she was. I assured her that He would. I also gave Kim the script she had just repeated to start the healing process. She needed to love herself as she began to nurture her inner child who had been abused and neglected.

Kim's ability to trust me and share led her to release anger. The work would advance her healing, yet I cautioned her to allow herself the time to heal.

Saltwater tip: Take time to love and heal your inner child.

Hero Story

Former ballet dancer Nasha Thomas, now in her fifties, is the national director of AileyCamp, an Alvin Ailey summer camp that shares the gift of dance with underserved young people. Instead of ending her career, she assumed a meaningful role with a focus on mentoring, which Nasha says is incredibly more fulfilling than performing.

John Bradshaw, author, television personality, and speaker who was known for promoting self-help by teaching adults to care for their damaged inner child, presented the following six stages of healing from past wounds in his book *Homecoming: Reclaiming and Championing Your Inner Child*:

1. Trust

For your wounded inner child to come out of hiding, she must be able to trust that you will be there for her. Your inner child also needs a supportive, non-shaming ally to validate her abandonment, neglect, abuse, and enmeshment. Those are the first essential elements in original pain work.

2. Validation

If you're still inclined to minimize and/or rationalize the ways in which you were shamed, ignored, or used to nurture your parents, you need now to accept the fact that these things truly wounded your soul. Your parents weren't bad; they were just wounded kids themselves.

3. Shock and Anger

If this is all shocking to you, that's great, because shock is the beginning of grief. It's okay to be angry, even if what was done to you was unintentional. In fact, you must be angry if you want to heal your wounded inner child. I don't mean you need to scream and holler, although you might. It's just okay to be mad about a dirty deal.

I know my parents did the best that two wounded adult children could do. But I'm also aware that I was deeply wounded spiritually and that it's had life-damaging consequences for me. What that means is that I hold us all responsible to stop what we're doing to ourselves and to others. I will not tolerate the outright dysfunction and abuse that dominated my family system.

4. Sadness

After anger comes hurt and sadness. If we were victimized, we must grieve that betrayal. We must also grieve what might've been—our dreams and aspirations. We must grieve our unfulfilled developmental needs.

5. Remorse

When we grieve for someone who's died, remorse is sometimes more relevant. For instance, perhaps we wish we'd spent more time with the deceased person. Grieving childhood abandonment, you must help your wounded inner child see that there was nothing she could've done differently. Her pain is about what happened to her; it's about the child who endured the abuse.

6. Loneliness

The deepest core feelings of grief are toxic shame and loneliness. We were shamed by our parents abandoning us. We feel we are bad, as if we're contaminated, and that shame leads to loneliness. Since our inner child feels flawed and defective, she must cover up her true self with her adapted, false self. She then comes to identify herself by her false self. Her true self remains alone and isolated.

Staying with this last layer of painful feelings is the hardest part of the grief process. "The only way out is through," we say in therapy. It's hard to stay at that level of shame and loneliness; but as we embrace these feelings, we come out the other side. We encounter the self that has been in hiding. Because we hid it from others, we hid it from ourselves. By embracing our shame and loneliness, we begin to touch our truest self.

The past is hard to look at; continuing to carry the pain is harder. At some point, the pain becomes too much. Kim not only had to heal from abuse, but also from abandonment. Even though her parents were there financially, they were not present for her emotionally and spiritually. They also neglected to protect her.

The Other Women

I lost touch with Luna when she moved away after leaving Dick. Carol and Jolinda, however, both stayed in touch with me. All in our fifties, we had the menopausal issues to deal with on top of our friend group going awry. Consequently, Carol, who had walked in on Kim and Dick, called me one afternoon. She didn't necessarily want an official therapy session but needed someone to talk to. I had great respect for Carol, who, by then, had all three of her homeschooled children in college.

It was a rainy, fall afternoon in Atlanta when Carol stepped into my foyer. She shook her umbrella, placed it in the corner, and I welcomed her with a hug and a cup of hot tea, her favorite drink. Joining us, my three Aussies, nestled on the floor, were sad because the rain was interfering with their ball-catching time. Carol and I discussed the Alpharetta dinner club briefly, and Kim was mentioned. Although I would never disclose confidential information, I assured Carol that healing was underway. That put a smile on her face.

Conscious of her need to talk, I asked, "Carol, what's going on?"

"Well, John and my sex life has not been great," she confided. "Don't get me wrong. I love him deeply, we have a great friendship, but our sex life has taken a major nosedive."

Going through perimenopause, she had picked up some weight and lost her drive completely.

"Oh, Carol," I said, "this is common for women our age. Tell me, is it more of a mental issue or is it more physical?"

"It's physical," she said. "It hurts."

Carol gave me a few more details, so I knew what she was struggling with: vaginal atrophy.

The Mayo Clinic provides the following information on the topic:

Vaginal atrophy (atrophic vaginitis) is thinning, drying and inflammation of the vaginal walls due to your body having less estrogen. Vaginal atrophy occurs most often after menopause.

For many women, vaginal atrophy not only makes intercourse painful, but also leads to distressing urinary symptoms. Because of the interconnected nature of the vaginal and urinary symptoms of this condition, experts agree that a more accurate term for vaginal atrophy and its accompanying symptoms is "genitourinary syndrome of menopause (GSM)."

Simple, effective treatments for genitourinary syndrome of menopause— vaginal atrophy and its urinary symptoms— are available. Reduced estrogen levels result in changes to your body, but it doesn't mean you have to live with the discomfort of GSM.

Symptoms
With moderate to severe genitourinary syndrome of meno-
pause (GSM), you may experience the following vaginal
and urinary signs and symptoms:
    Vaginal dryness
    Vaginal burning
    Vaginal discharge
    Genital itching
    Burning with urination
    Urgency with urination
    More urinary tract infections
    Urinary incontinence
    Light bleeding after intercourse
    Discomfort with intercourse
    Decreased vaginal lubrication during sexual activity
    Shortening and tightening of the vaginal canal

Many women, too embarrassed to tell their doctors, remain silent about the issue, and the problem affects countless marriages. Studies indicate up to sixty percent of menopausal women are affected.

Remedies for vaginal atrophy include the following:

- Using a vaginal moisturizer regularly to help moisten and re-estrogenize the vaginal walls

- Having more sex! Regular sexual activity, with or without a partner, can help maintain healthy vaginal tissues.

Telling Carol that I was delighted she'd shared and that John would be glad as well, I recommended Amata Life Vaginal Moisturizer, a product of Dr. Christiane Northrup. Find details in the resources listed in the back of this book.

"Now, honey," I advised Carol, "you go buy it and try it, and call me and let me know! I'm sure this is what you need!

We giggled like two school girls, and I shared how my sex drive had hit rock bottom as my weight soared, too.

"Then I found Amata Life and wow!" I exclaimed. "Oh, yeah, it's hot around the Teague home again—sizzling hot, two to three times a week, yeah, baby! Jeff is a happy camper these days."

I told Carol that Jeff had struggled with me through this. A gentle man, he was willing to wait for me to straighten it out. Also, Jeff and I have a strong friendship and that carried us.

Talking to the husbands, I will say that right after a woman has a baby, for instance, you have to wait patiently. Another of those times can be when she's making the passage into menopause. Many women experience their sex drive diminishing as estrogen drops. It will reach a stable level, and if you're patient and understanding, you'll be dancing and burning off the midnight oil again before you know it.

I further reminded Carol to have her doctor check her vitamin D levels, which can affect libido. You need 4,000 to 5,000 IUs (international units) per day. Sunlight is a great source, but often not sufficient.

Although I made Carol blush to a deep shade of red when I told her that she and John would be rolling around under the sheets again soon, more than anything I wanted them to be happy and healthy in their marriage.

Salt Water Tip #: For vaginal atrophy, try Amata Life Vaginal Moisturizer and check vitamin D levels.

Soon after Carol's visit, Jolinda and I had a lunch date at our favorite tea room in Alpharetta. From celebrating my daughter's fifth birthday there, I had fond memories of the little five-year-old girls dancing around in their princess gowns. Entering the establishment, I had to push down a lump in my throat. I couldn't believe my baby girl was in college! Seeing Jolinda, an inspiring woman with a heart of gold and a full calendar, however, always put a smile on my face. The social butterfly of the group, she'd always throw the best parties—fun with many new people to get to know. I've always said that Jolinda is a collector of friends. Hugging, we began chatting, stopping momentarily to order our favorite sandwiches.

Suddenly, Jolinda looked at me and took a deep sigh.

"What's wrong?" I asked.

"I'm burned out!" she blurted. "My get-up-and-go has gotten up and left. I'm just not myself lately.

I encouraged her to tell me more, and our lunch hour continued for three hours. Jolinda described a lack of sleep, moodiness, and outbursts at her husband. The behavior did not at all reflect her usual temperament. When I mentioned anxiety and depression, she was surprised, but fatigue—a big factor in the equation—was a sure sign. Jolinda was not sleeping.

Staying Level-Headed

Maintaining a sense of sanity during so many bodily and life changes may seem impossible, but taking control yields great benefits. In addition to having your doctor test you for a hormonal imbalance, consider my suggestions for remaining level headed during this time.

1. Rhythmic Breathing

Lowering your stress response is the first step to clearing your head, and one of the best ways to do this is through practicing rhythmic breathing. Focusing solely on producing slow, conscious, and mindful breaths for around ten to fifteen minutes a day helps reduce heart rate, blood pressure, and respiration rate. The physical changes in your body result in a better sense of well-being and will clear your mind, leaving it free to think of solutions to possible problems instead of being overwhelmed by them.

2. Regular Exercise

Regular exercise also helps reduce the amount of stress that can build up during menopause, and thus keep you level-headed. With physical activity comes the production of endorphins, and this can increase sense of well-being and elevate mood. In addition, exercise can also reduce the effects of menopause symptoms, such as hot flashes. Minimizing them can lift your mood if they are getting you down.

3. Valerian Herbal Supplement

Although incorporating exercise and rhythmic breathing can be excellent long-term remedies against feeling low during menopause, it can sometimes help increase motivation if you take an herbal remedy to increase mood for a few weeks. Although valerian is not recommended to be taken for more than a few weeks at any one time, it naturally promotes relaxation and could give you a kickstart.

Among all other recommendations, I reminded Jolinda to stay present in the moment and enjoy the simple things in life. I gave her an example of how I'd taken my own advice in going back to doing something I'd always loved: planting petunias and other flowers. Nurturing my plants, I told her, gave me great joy and reminded me of what was important. The following story perfectly illustrated my point:

135

One July evening, after experiencing two busy weeks and losing track of watering the potted plants on my deck, I saw that some of my favorite flowers had shriveled up to nothing but a dried-out root system and some brownish stems. I poured water into the sad pot before tending to the other plants that had survived the drought. When I returned to the deck the next morning, to my surprise, I noticed that the seemingly dead stems had plumped up. Within the week, green leaves were coming back out and buds were forming. Two weeks later, I had beautiful purple and violet blossoms. The plant survived well into the fall and the first cold days. There was something healing and empowering about watching that plant come back. The rebirth and growth signified what Jolinda and I were experiencing in becoming empty-nesters and shifting our focus to a new season.

Recalling my conversation with Jolinda on the ride home, I thought about how my Aussies how been so wonderful and loving to have at home. Pets of any kind can be a great source of joy during the many seasons of life. Similarly, birdwatching from my deck is another pleasure of mine, and my husband and kids had surprised me on Mother's Day by making me three beautiful bird houses. Taking their time, they had handmade and painted each one in bright colors. I love watching the bluebirds come and nest in them each spring and summer. What a special gift! Enticing other species, I also hung a hummingbird feeder.

Enjoying God's creations brings great pleasure, especially during this time of physical change. Find the simple things and enjoy them!

CHAPTER NINE

Finding What Works for You

**"You have to love yourself because no amount of
love from others is sufficient to fill the yearning
that your soul requires from you."
Dodinsky**

"I feel horrible. I'm angry all the time," Cheryl confessed.

She had become especially irritable and snappy with her
children. She'd even become irate over a simple question
from her son to find his shoes. Normally Cheryl would have
scoured the house, searching diligently until they were found.
Now she found herself hostile in responding and barking back
in an ugly tone, "I don't know! You find them."

Cheryl felt resentful over duties such as working full-time
and doing all the household chores, including all the shopping
and cooking, coordinating and providing rides to all the kids

extra-curricular activities without her husband's help. "Okay, Cheryl, you are Superwoman," we would chuckle. She managed everything so well for years—until the effort became unbearable. She resented her husband and the children, while feeling guilty. A stew pot of mixed emotions, the resentment spewed over the top, escalating into arguments and shouting matches with her husband.

Cheryl also started feeling paranoid. She felt like she could not trust her husband who had faithfully been there throughout the years. She felt suspicious of his motives. She began listening in on his conversations, as if searching for a reason to say, I knew it! She had a growing suspicion that he was talking about her behind her back. The paranoia worsened to the point that she accused her best friend of excluding her and talking about her behind her back.

Hero Story

Carmen Kluckhohn retired from her profession as an elementary school teacher to become a cyclist. Rather than stick to her neighborhood, however, Carmen, who is in her fifties, travels the world. While building physical and mental endurance, she is exploring and forging new friendships.

As Cheryl and I continued to discuss what was going on, I was able to show her that her perceptions were off. Finally, she could see that her husband and her best friend had not changed at all. She described having persistent, unwanted suspicions, thoughts and feelings. She oscillated from paranoia and mistrust to resentment and anger, and then back. She also complained of hot flashes and night sweats and difficulty sleeping.

Cheryl decided to go with a homeopathic approach.

If you choose that route, the upcoming chart from the National Center for Homeopathy may help you to guide your doctor or homeopath in the right direction. (It helps tremendously to be able to tell them exactly what is going on with your symptoms.) I am neither a doctor nor a homeopath, so please check with these professionals before adding these to your supplements. **Note: do not do this without a homeopath professional.**

The Homeopathic Approach

Prescribing guidelines

- Take the selected remedy in a low potency (6C, 30X or 30C).

- Repeat the remedy 2-4 times a day according to the seriousness of your symptoms (less serious, less often; more serious more often).

- Stop taking it as soon you notice an improvement. A homeopathic medicine acts as a catalyst, stimulating the body to heal itself. You only need take the "minimum" dose or amount needed to stimulate that healing response.

- If the same symptoms return then repeat the same remedy—starting and stopping—until there is more lasting improvement.

- If you have taken a remedy for 3-5 days with no improvement then it is probably the wrong one. Select a different remedy and/or seek professional help.

- If you have had a constitutional remedy prescribed by your homeopath within the past 6 months, check with them first before taking any remedies to treat your symptoms yourself.

Amylenum nitrosum	Tremendous anxiety felt in head & chest Feels like something bad is going to happen	Severe hot flashes: head is hot; face flushes (deep red) Drenching sweats after hot flash	Palpitations and headaches. Sensation of a lump in the throat Exhaustion after a hot flash (with the sweating)	Craves fresh air (opens window in coldest weather)
Argentum nitricum	Tremendous anxiety (constant agitation) Many fears including heights, crowds; doesn't go out	Severe hot flashes with sudden, drenching sweats	Insomnia with agitation: gets overheated, flings covers off and then gets chilled	Worse for heat Craves sweets which aggravate
Belladonna	Sensitive and excitable Intense Restless: especially in bed (with flashes)	Severe hot flashes: head is boiling hot, hands/ feet are icy cold; with profuse sweats (or none) Bright red flush spreads over face	Stress incontinence when walking/ standing Throbbing headaches, nosebleeds. Menstrual flooding. Insomnia with twitching, jerking, grinding teeth, hot flashes	Symptoms come on strongly and suddenly Tendency to dryness

Calcarea carbonica	Anxious about her health Confused Difficulty concentrating Memory weak	none) Bright red flush spreads over face Hot flashes: with tremendous heat; with drenching sweats; followed by chills and clamminess Sweats mostly on head & feet	Yeast infections with itching/ burning discharges Headaches with dizziness. Menstrual flooding Strains joints easily especially ankles Cramps in calves at night	Sluggish: energy low Metabolism slows; gains weight easily Worse cold/ damp and drafts
China officionalis	Depressed & apathetic Full of ideas but doesn't want to do anything	Hot flashes day & night Sweats when covered	Menstrual flooding with anemia and exhaustion Throbbing headaches	Face pale. Chilly and faint Absolutely exhausted
Cimicifuga racemosa	Black depression alternating with excitability		Menstrual flooding: with chilliness and exhaustion: periods are painful and more frequent than usual Pains in the small joints (in the feet/ hands/ wrists etc.)	Changeable symptoms Pains that move from place to place

Glonoinum	Gets lost easily (even in familiar places) Scared when out and about	Frequent severe hot flashes with nausea, dizziness & faint feeling Flushes rush up or down the body	Violent palpitations felt in whole body, even in fingertips Heat & pressure felt in head. Hot sensation down the back Clothes feel tight	Worse for heat. Worse for wine. Better for fresh air and anything cool
Ignatia	A sense of loss. Keeps feelings to self. Sighs a lot. Moods changeable: alternate between irritability, laughing and even crying.	Hot flashes: with headache; with sweating on the face especially	Sleeps lightly & easily disturbed Emptiness in stomach no better for eating	Contradictory symptoms Worse for coffee
Lachesis	Mood swings: depressed to irritable to anxious. Wound up over little things Much worse in the mornings on waking	Hot flashes felt in whole body Sleep disturbed by hot flashes (woken by them)—no sweating	Severe, left-sided headaches. Menstrual flooding Bloating and discomfort after eating Cannot tolerate tight clothing especially around neck	Everything is worse in the morning on waking Worse for heat & coffee

Lycopodium	Irritable, depressed and anxious	Hot flashes: worse when anxious; worse in stuffy places; with clammy sweat and red face—clothes feel too tight then	Sleep disturbed by jerking or restless legs Appetite disturbed; full after eating a little; lots of gas Hair loss. Menstrual flooding. Headache: vice-like pain	Worse 4-8 pm Craves sweets and chocolate
Natrum muriaticum	Depressed and withdrawn Great sense of loss; keeps it all to self Dwells on new and old resentments or hurts	Hot flashes that rise from chest to head (legs are cool) With night sweats and fluid retention	Dry skin generally; Lips dry, cracked Painful dryness of vagina; recurring yeast infections Herpes at corners of mouth. Constipated with small, hard stools	Worse for heat and sun Better when alone
Nux vomica	Irritable, oversensitive workaholics. Tend to overdo everything bad (alcohol, coffee, fat) and underdo good (exercise, fruits, veggies)	Hot flashes with profuse sweats that are worse in bed Feels faint with hot flash and sleepy afterwards	Insomnia: from anxious thoughts (about work); hot flashes; indigestion Headache: burning pain on top of the head Periods more frequent and heavier (flooding)	Extremely chilly (hates drafts)

143

Pulsatilla	Extremely moody: sensitive, easily upset, weepy Generally better for company and affection	Hot flashes, waves of heat with blushing (face and neck) and night sweats	Frequent urination and stress incontinence Joint pains that move about the body Headaches and digestive problems after rich/ fatty foods	Better for fresh air Worse for stuffy rooms Thirstless
Sepia	Depressed, apathetic (not interested in anything) Irritable— snaps at loved ones (or anyone) Weepy: doesn't want company or sympathy	Hot flashes followed by drenching sweats— moving up the body with exhaustion	Dragging down sensation in lower abdomen/ lower back Dry painful vagina and recurring yeast infections Stress incontinence	Worse for cold Better for vigorous exercise
Sulphur	Depressed and weepy Becomes or feels cut off from people	Hot flashes with painful, burning heat at top of head. With faint feeling Burning heat of hands/feet. Uncovers feet	Nosebleeds. Menstrual flooding. Hemorrhoids after periods stop Insomnia— restless with the flashes. Dry, itchy skin	Worse for heat Better for cool fresh air Very thirsty

One month after the homeopathic visit, Cheryl's hot flashes and sweats had completely disappeared, and she was sleeping a great deal better. She still experienced some irritability, but it had lessened.

Cheryl also addressed her unresolved emotional issues. She had stayed so busy being Superwoman that she had tucked her own emotional needs under the carpet and kept moving until the shift into perimenopause caused all her emotional needs to surface.

Her extreme paranoia prompted me to suggest that she see a licensed psychologist. I love walking alongside Cheryl as her friend and counselor, yet I felt a little more monitoring was necessary. Cheryl continued to feel much better, and her paranoia did eventually roll off. She needed to surround herself with people who cared enough to see the real issues, and I'm glad she chose to do that.

If you are dealing with extreme paranoia, please get professional help and know you do not have to live with your quality and sense of well-being robbed. Help is available. As you learn to love and care for yourself, please consider additional items that may help you.

Self-love Checklist for Perimenopausal and Menopausal Women

Self-love applies to each and every being on the planet, regardless of race, gender, religion or culture. In this season of change, when physical (hormonal), mental, and emotional change are all inevitable, you must practice balance. If you don't, you may suffer depression, bitterness, anxiety, resentment, and grief. Without first learning how to love yourself, how can you truly know how to love others? I think of a reservoir verses a canal as an analogy.

"A canal spreads abroad water as it receives it, but a reservoir waits until it is filled before overflowing, and thus without loss to itself [it shares] its superabundant water."
—Bernard of Clairvaux

A rich illustration of the canal is one that runs dry so quickly, shortly after the rains stop, becoming parched dry mud and sand. Imagine a dry streambed in the desert. But a reservoir represents vast, deep reserves like a heart full of life!

You are called to live in a way in which you store up reserves in your life and heart, and only then can you offer from a place of abundance. As you have learned self-love, you will master this in a big way. Oh, what a rich deep life you have when you are full and nurtured and cherishing yourself! From this abundance, you pour out into your family, friends and the community.

It is impossible for you to give love if you haven't first filled yourself. I see women give and give and give to the point of throwing themselves out of balance. When this season of perimenopause comes, they don't have the reserves—what they need for themselves—to make it through. The key is slowing down and tending to yourself.

Twenty-one Ways to Practice Self-Love

1. **Begin each day with prayer and meditation.** Recognize there is a God of the Universe running the show. Shift into gratitude for all your blessings. Acknowledging God and your blessings each day changes your countenance.

2. **Treat yourself like you would your best friend.** It's easy to become your worst mortal enemy. To heal yourself, you must change your relationship with yourself consciously; treat yourself with compassion and consideration just as you would with a best friend.

146

3. **Identify your negative thinking patterns.** Within all of us, subtle and incessant voices sabotage and paralyze us. Cultivating self-awareness through practices such as mindfulness meditation or stop-think exercises and focusing on the positive are key to overcoming negative self-talk. Remember, you are loved, cherished, and adored.

4. **Get seven to eight hours of sleep every night.** Getting less than the recommended hours of sleep every night lowers your immunity and contributes to chronic fatigue, moodiness, depression, anxiety issues, chronic pain, and fibromyalgia. Also, set a stable bedtime. Aim to go to bed around 10:00 p.m. and rise at 6:00 a.m. Some schedules will not allow for this, but do your best to get an ideal amount of sleep. You will feel the difference mentally and emotionally!

5. **Learn quiet assertiveness.** Being obnoxious is not necessary. Knowing how to stand up for yourself and setting healthy boundaries are vital. Remember *Horton Hears a Who*? You are here! Stand up for yourself and do not feel guilty.

6. **Explore your mental traps.** Low self-esteem is often a result of false and unrealistic thought patterns that are deeply ingrained. Such patterns may be composed of mental traps, such as assumptions, beliefs, comparisons, desires, expectations, and ideals about yourself and others. One great way to explore your mental traps is by keeping a daily diary of your private thoughts and feelings. Keeping a dream journal is vital. You may, for instance, dream about key ideas, events, and past occurrences, and reviewing them can lead to healing, growth, and soul care.

7. **Eat a nutritious diet.** Getting sugary, processed foods out of your diet will make you feel wonderful about yourself.

Revisit Chapter 3 on lifestyle changes that revolve around eating.

8. **Welcome solitude into your life.** When you don't make space in your life to be alone, you will find it's easier to burn out, become disorientated, even ill. Each day, make time for yourself to unwind, relax, and reflect—alone. Solitude provides insight and perspective. It reinstates harmony in your life. I regularly see women overextend themselves and suffer burnout as a result. By nature, you are a nurturer, lover, and giver, and you must maintain a balance in this season between pouring out to others and pouring back to yourself.

9. **Identify the toxic people in your life.** They are the ones who make you feel wretched and significantly lower the quality of your daily life. Toxic people are often judgmental, manipulative, clingy, backstabbing, ruthless, aggressive, controlling, deceitful, self-pitying, and self-destructive. While it's important to learn that such people act out from a place of pain, it's also vital to take care of yourself. Learning to cut away those who hinder your self-growth can be difficult, but the step is necessary on your journey of healing. If they are family members, learn to set healthy boundaries. In doing so, you will feel better, and they will learn to treat you better with time.

10. **Seek supportive companions.** Supportive people encourage you, uplift you, and inspire you. They have often obtained a high level of self-love, and because of their ability to respect themselves, they can easily respect and love others. You may not have to seek out such people; instead, you gravitate towards them. Making the effort to instigate friendships and connections with supportive companions will help you during dark periods.

11. **Learn to trust your intuition**. Your unconscious mind is an ocean of wisdom, understanding, and insight. Intuition—that mysterious inner guide you have—is a manifestation of this vast, untapped world within you. Learning to trust your intuition will help you to live a life that's true to yourself and your deepest needs.

12. **Take a walk or jog each day.** Even if walking or jogging is not always possible, regular exercise has an immense benefit on your body, mind, and soul, proving that you are actively taking care of yourself. Getting moving and fight being sedentary.

13. **Stop spending so much time on social networks.** Did you know that average American adults check their social media accounts at least once every waking hour of the day? In total, that equals about four or more hours each day spent on websites and apps such as Facebook, Twitter, Snapchat, Instagram, and Pinterest. The number is also increasing. A great deal of science has been used to respond to likes, shares, followers, and friends because of social acceptance and esteem. The environment can be highly detrimental to your health, even causing depression and low self-esteem. Try turning off and unplugging your digital devices regularly and opting for real-world interaction.

14. **Reassess your wardrobe.** Colors impact your psyche. People who replace their black, gray and dull-colored clothing with brighter alternatives notice an interesting difference in their mental states. Wearing light blue stimulates feelings of openness, and yellow boosts optimism. Drab colors like khaki, granite, and charcoal are all associated with feelings of apathy, aloofness, pessimism, and despondency. Also, wearing pretty jewelry with interesting stones and colors can be fun for you, and you may find

your brighter look and attitude are compelling more people to strike up conversations with you. More positive interactions will add more fun to your day.

15. **Make time to explore your passion.** What drives you, fires you up, fills you with a sense of accomplishment? When you only feed your need to cater to others' needs, you may lose sight of what truly makes you happy in life. Many abandon dreams at an early age; instead, they live meaningless lives of drudgery and socially approved pursuits—i.e., having a good career, big house, nice car, perfect family, etc. You must ask: What is my passion? Remember that passions evolve with you; they are not static. Whether painting, writing, dancing, designing, building, or whatever it is excites you, pursue it, even if as something you enjoy observing.

16. **Focus on reducing sources of stress in your life.** Prolonged stress contributes to so many illnesses. Stress can be reduced by dropping your desires and expectations for yourself, others, and situations in life. You may also minimize stress by practicing many of the suggestions I have presented previously: diet, exercise, soul care, and spiritual exercises.

17. **Accept your flaws and celebrate your strengths.** Come to terms with the fact that you are imperfect. There is no denying it. By accepting your flaws, you open the doorway to self-improvement. Embrace your warts and pimples. Don't run away from them. Learn how to celebrate your strengths. Keep a journal of affirmations and each day list every little thing you appreciate about yourself.

18. **Accept rather than punish yourself.** Does a good friend punish you with an onslaught of verbal criticism for hours? No! A true friend accepts both the good and bad in you without passing vicious judgment. A true friend realizes

that no one is perfect, and everyone has a "monster," whether large or small, within them. Be a true friend to yourself. Not only is acceptance the healthier option, but it also opens doorways that allow you to solve your problems, not wallow in them.

19. **Learn to laugh at yourself.** Now, don't laugh in a scornful manner of ridicule, but as a friend would laugh *with* you. Be good-natured toward yourself and find humor in the quirky little things you say, think, and do. When you stop taking yourself so seriously, you open yourself up to more inner harmony and wholeness. A lightness will fill the atmosphere around you, and your friends and family will notice. Trust me, there will be lots to laugh about! (Think of my crossing that stone bridge on the golf course in my car!)

20. **Realize that you are SO worthy.** If you equate failure in your life with personally being a failure, remember that if you outsource your self-worth and self-esteem, you will always wind up feeling like a miserable failure. Why? The thoughts, opinions, beliefs and expectations that you use as yardsticks to measure your success and worth are outside your control. They constantly fluctuate and change, perhaps causing you to feel like a failure because you never cultivated an inner and innate sense of worthiness.

21. **Learn how to support and comfort yourself.** Many of us drown out our pain by indulging in food, sex, gambling, and other addictions with the added harms of self-pity and other self-destructive behaviors. Learning how to face your hurt, instead of escaping from it, is one of the most essential and most difficult ways of developing self-love. When you listen to your emotional needs and open yourself to the vulnerability of experiencing shame, anger, and grief, you can then take the appropriate steps to help quench the

hurt you feel in a healthy and productive way. Self-love is complete forgiveness, acceptance, and respect for who you are deep down—including perceived hideous parts. When you love yourself, you take care of yourself, honor your limitations, listen to your needs, and respect your dreams enough to act on them. When you love yourself, your happiness, health, and fulfillment are all important because you realize that without loving yourself, you will never be able to love others genuinely.

Now, give yourself a big hug and say out loud: I love, honor and accept myself!

Practicing some or all of the checklist behaviors daily will change your perspective and empower you to be an empowered woman of love, beauty, and honor. As you make the menopausal passage, think of the ocean. Imagine the waves roaring and pouring in and then pulling back. Take a deep breath and let this season in and then let the breath out. Breathe while doing an inventory of the way you have navigated life. Have you loved yourself, have you loved others? What are your goals from this point forward?

Perimenopause was a frightening and lonely time for me, yet I would not trade this season because of the great lessons learned. I'm speaking to all of you who are reading this and are experiencing this lonely confusion. As you look within, become a good detective on what your body and soul need.

We've covered hormones and symptoms, we've covered ways to change your diet to assist in healing and wholeness, including supplements, and we've looked at many prayer patterns and tools such as Tapping and inner-child work. Before we move into the last chapter of this book, I want to highlight finding your Tribe. Your tribe is a group of like-minded people who fuel your calling and your passion. Isolation in this season is deadly! That's a strong word, I know, and I mean it. Finding your tribe is critical because, as you can see with the women I counsel, this season is a time for unresolved issues to rise to the top.

The onset of perimenopause triggers the process of reclaiming personal power. "Any uncomfortable symptoms that reveal themselves during times of hormonal shifts will be magnified and prolonged if a woman is carrying a heavy load of emotional baggage," explains Christiane Northrup, M.D., in her book *The Wisdom of Menopause.* She goes on to explain that while our culture leads us to believe that our mood swings are a result of raging hormones, the opposite is true. Evidence shows that repeated episodes of stress due to relationships, children, job situation, or any life issue you feel powerless over, are behind many of the hormonal changes in the brain and body. All unresolved issues, stemming from childhood and perpetuating in every subsequent relationship, are contributing to, and exacerbating, the perimenopausal hormonal imbalance.

The Wisdom of Menopause further explains how the body sends us continuous signals to look within. The changes in brain chemistry issue a wake-up call to heal body, mind, and emotions. The first of the series of wake-up calls happens during PMS, as the monthly reminder of the growing backlog of unresolved issues accumulating within. Since women's brains are hormonally programmed to nurture others at the expense of the self, their grievances often get swept under the carpet during the childbearing years.

In this season, you must tend to yourself by loving and nurturing uourself and doing the work to get old and unresolved issues healed. What makes or breaks this work is often the people with whom you surround yourself.

Some people give off positive energy that makes you feel good. You probably have that friend you just love being with because your cup is full after you are with that person. Unfortunately, you can possibly think of someone who gives off negative energy and drains you. When you see her name come up on your cell, you dread taking the call. Yeah, that's the one! Take note. Pay attention to the signals that your intuition sends you and act on them. Let your intuition lead you to a healthy social network.

The following checklist will confirm your intuition:

- Does your conversation flow easily, or is it filled with dread and a forced effort to share?

- Do you feel truly understood, supported, and accepted?

- Do you also truly understand, support, and accept them?

- Do you feel better or worse about yourself after spending time with them?

- Do you leave them feeling full and energized or despondent and mildly depressed?

- Do you include them in your life for fulfillment and intimacy, or are they just filling a void in your life, giving you the feeling that you have a friend?

Answering the questions can help you assess your friendships and begin to know who should stay and who should go, or with whom to set boundaries. Developing intuition will strengthen your relationships or help you with letting them go, if necessary.

Remember, it is okay to admit your vulnerability and ask for help. Doing so is a strength! It just needs to be with the right people. When you find those treasured friendships, you will be available to them and they will be available to you. They are your jewels! Keep them!

At times, you will recognize that someone in your life is no longer good for you. It is fine to let that person go. If you would like to keep the individual in your life out of loyalty, you can stay in touch, but remember that the person is not the one you can count on for support. Keeping the person at bay and in a peripheral role might serve you well. Just remember that this one is not able to give you the support you deserve. Only you can decide if the relationship is worth keeping or not.

Having several people whom you can count on in life is important. While cultivating a circle of loving and supportive friends, who often become like family, takes some work, the effort does make a huge difference in how you handle stress and life.

Not everyone will be a part of your tribe. If someone in your life constantly makes you feel bad, doesn't share the same interest or values, or clashes with you, it is perfectly acceptable to put the relationship on the back-burner. Letting a relationship fade or not develop comes with important lessons that you must learn. Seasons change, and people change, so you may sometimes grow in different directions. That's okay. It does not mean that something is wrong with either of you. You simply accept that the season is over.

I like to look at such changes as going from 2-D to 3-D. A 3-D movie has so much more depth and richness than a 2-D movie. Was the 2-D movie good? Of course! However, when you see it in 3-D, you delight at the depth and richness, catching many details that were, perhaps, left out before. Forming an inner tribe of 3-D friendships is life-changing.

Keep your 2-D friends on the outer circle.

May we all have a huge 3-D tribe of close friends!

Saltwater Tip: Decipher emotional support vs. hormonal support, knowing that you need both. You must love yourself first before extending it to others. Assessing your tribe is critical for support.

CHAPTER TEN

Love Rising

**"Do everything with gentleness, with kindness,
with reverence. That is how grace moves;
that is how love dances."**
Heather K. O'Hare

The crisp fall air in October was amazing! Georgia always has a beautiful autumn, especially north towards the mountains. It would be the ideal time to visit Barefoot Ranch. After our horseback riding retreat to Barefoot Ranch in the spring went so well that we—the ladies whom I counsel and I—decided to return there. Along for the trip were two van-loads of women from an Atlanta homeless shelter. We were all excited that Adrienne could attend this time, too, as our prior visit has been scheduled just before her mastectomy. Thankfully, she was doing well.

Barefoot Ranch is a rescue facility for horses, and my charity is a rescue for prostitutes and destitute women who find themselves in dire straits. It's a place of healing laughter and great adventures. The horses instinctively seemed to know that the ladies in my group were hurting. I'll never forget how a horse reached its neck around one of the women as if hugging her in a huge welcome.

Darrith, who runs the ranch, loaded us all up on horses with the instruction to ride them down to the ring where she would give the lesson. While we were all steering our horses into the ring and waiting on Darrith, I gently nudged my horse with the back of my heel. The horse went from zero to sixty miles an hour! I have no idea how I hung on, but my butt was glued to the seat of that saddle. Even though my transportation bucked and jumped and went wild, I did not bite the dust! I should probably thank Darrith, who caught up with us.

"Pull in the reins! Pull . . . in . . . the . . . reins!" she screamed.

I finally did, and the horse came to a halt.

"Okay, ladies," Darrith announced, "we are starting the day out with a pow punch!"
Everyone was in hysterics.

A worker from the ranch ran up to the fence and asked, "Who is that lady?" After one of the homeless women identified me as the person who ran the charity, he said, "Okay! Wow! Ride 'em, cowgirl!"

"It must be the Cherokee Indian blood I have," I declared.

After I got my adrenaline back under control and carefully kept my feet in the stirrups, we all headed out for two hours on the trail. It was two hours of sheer bliss. There was something so healing about being in nature and sharing the experience in the mountains—beautiful, gentle giants. The day culminated with a cookout and music at the ranch. My daughter played guitar and sang several special songs she had written for the ladies. After, she shared some good 'ole campfire songs, and we all sang along. Perfect icing on the cake for a heartfelt day! The setting sun signaled the time for the ladies from the shelter to return to Atlanta, and hugging each, I choked back a lump in my throat. Many had suffered so much, and I'd been honored to serve as an agent of love and healing in their lives. Only by God's grace have I been able to do the work I do: I stood in their shoes many, many moons ago. By God's grace, another woman had reached out to me in love, telling me, "here's hope," and taking me. I stayed with her for a season, until I could get back on my feet. I've simply returned the same that was done for me.

We all can agree that grace has a mysterious nature.

Just as you can hear the wind but can't tell where it comes from or where it will go next, so it is with the Spirit. (John 3:8)

Throughout this book, I've shared journeys of courageous ladies. Each will tell you that spiritual growth and healing are not an orderly, predictable process. As you seek and grow, there will be stumbling blocks along the way. The key is to pick up and continue to move forward and remain open to the miraculous coming of grace. As you prepare your heart to be fertile ground for seeds of love, the miraculous does happen. I see it every time! It's amazing what happens when someone is cherished, tended too, poured into, and loved!

Saltwater Tip: Love sets the stage for the miraculous. That's why it's called amazing grace!

New Pathways

As we come to the end of our sessions and counseling, I often host a dinner party to which I invite all the ladies. I ask each to bring something that has a significant meaning about her counseling journey and to wrap it attractively as a gift. It could be a picture, a trinket, or anything. Each knows she'll tell why it's significant and then give it away.

I typically feel like I'm fluttering through the house when making final preparations for this dinner. Such times of sharing and connecting are among my favorites. I'm certain I'll be in touch with the attendees, but not in the same way. Either the session, the season, or the intensity is ending, but I encourage everyone to find a tribe—but a like-minded tribe—and stay in community. Staying in community—sharing and connecting on a deep soul level—is vital to well-being. Many opportunities exist to do this, such as running groups, gyms, churches, and civic groups, and I recommend options that fuel your passion and your soul!

Also, I encourage each one to step outside her normal routine.

The advice reminds me of my son's first year of driving. We'd bought Josh a shiny, red jeep for his sixteenth birthday, and it wasn't long before I picked up my cell to hear he'd gone off an embankment to avoid hitting another vehicle. I'll never forget the panic I felt in my chest. Incredibly, Josh was completely unharmed. God definitely had His watchful eye on him.

As grateful as we were, the incident forced me back on the schedule of carpooling the kids to school. I drove them in a box—to school, to practice, to drama, and home again—for ten years. My reference to a box wasn't about the car; it described the unchanged, rectangular route I took over the same roads.

In the short four months Josh had been driving, he'd found all sorts of shortcuts. One morning in route to school, he said, "Mom, you waste so much time driving this way."

"What do you mean?" I asked.

He said, "Turn here . . . and here . . . and here."

He proceeded to show me so many little back roads, and I felt a nudge, a spiritual nudge, that whispered in my ear: he is showing you a new way!

New pathways are right before your very eyes. What a picture of your journeys! New pathways are opening right before you, if you only take time to notice. Pause, pray, and ask God to give you a spiritual perspective. Step outside the natural and put on your spiritual eyes. Look with an eternal perspective.

A Special Dinner Party

I wasn't sure about the dynamics of the group this time, as three were from the original Alpharetta Dinner Club. However, everyone invited had connected at Barefoot Ranch, so I felt the group would work. Connections existed among all, so I trusted a gut feeling and went forward with it. Of course, my company-loving Aussies were going wild, welcoming everyone.

Shani, who happened to be in town for the weekend, showed up first. Like the others, she made a point of bringing an attractively wrapped gift. Jacelyn and Rainey showed up next, followed by Carol, Kim and Jolinda. Waiting another five minutes and anxious to bless everyone with dinner, I finally met Terri and Adrienne at the door. Eight in total had arrived, and I loved that we had eight—a number that represents new beginnings. How beautiful and prophetic!

We gathered around my circular dining room table for a delicious meal of sea bass and homemade Key lime pie, all prepared by Jeff. My husband, who missed his second calling as a chef, outdid himself. Our conversation remained light during dinner, after which Jeff poured everyone coffee and disappeared into the basement with our fur babies. It was time to exchange our significant gifts by drawing names.

Jolinda went first. She drew Kim's name, so Kim would present her gift to Jolinda. Unwrapping it carefully, she held up a plaque of a tree, engraved with the word *Wholeness*.

Almost choking up, I asked Kim to explain what it had meant to her, although I knew that she'd been working hard to heal and become whole.

"I'm so grateful for my healing journey," she said, "and I'm coming to realize how important it is that we become whole. The little pieces and fragments of my abuse are healing and integrating; it's a journey, and this represents my healing journey. I found the tree at an artsy craft store up in Dahlonega when I visited my son at college. It's for all women to heal."

Hugs and tissues went around the room, and then Adrienne drew Rainey's name. Rainey had brought a stone inscribed with the word *Courage*. How appropriate for Adrienne to draw a gift about courage! We were all proud of her fight against cancer. If you or anyone you know is fighting the disease, stand strong and fight! Know that invisible forces are linking up to fight your battle. God is with you!

Rainey had attached a note that said, "Courage doesn't always roar. Sometimes courage is that quiet voice at the end of the day, saying, I will try again tomorrow."

Rainey offered, "I found this stone in a store with my children while shopping. It just seemed to scream *pick me* at a time when it took a lot of courage to keep going with my charity. There was so much coming against my husband and me. I would keep that stone on me in a pocket or in my purse, and when it got tough, I'd pull it out and remember to keep going. My message is for all woman to take courage and move your mountains. God's grace will follow you as you stay clear to your passion and inner voice."

Notably, Rainey's nonprofit was still going strong.
Terri drew Carol, who presented her a sparkly gold package.

The pendant inside was engraved with a message: "God didn't bring me this far to leave me." Phil 1:6

After enduring a tumultuous couple of years in perimenopause, her hormones were returning to normal. Her marriage had also suffered, but by God's grace and their mutual love and understanding, they worked it out.

> Looking towards Terri, Carol said, "God brought me through, and He's bringing us all through each and every year."

Jacelyn then presented her gift to Kim. It was a plaque with a quote from Lord Byron: "Love will find a way through paths where wolves fear to prey." She had remarried after a horrible divorce, and her children were beginning to see the truth that the failed marriage was not all her fault.

> Conveying what the item had meant to her, Jacelyn said, "Losing my firm and marriage all within a two-year period was unbearable. One afternoon, I was wandering around The Avenues, killing some time, when I saw this in the window of a trendy store. I knew it was a message for me that things would turn around. Shortly after that, I met Sam, my new husband. Love found a way!"

She had not only managed to land with her feet firmly planted, but also gained a deeper faith in God. She displayed a new-found depth. While she would not wish her trials on anyone, Jacelyn was grateful to have acquired a bigger, softer heart, full of love!

Shani then gave Carol her gift, an artistic drawing of the earth with hands of all races holding it up and the Hebrew words *Tikkun Olam*. The phrase, found in the Mishnah, a body of classical rabbinic teachings, conveys that the importance of performing acts of kindness to perfect or repair the world.

It's a call to social action and social justice. Shani, who was directing children's musicals in another city and, taking my suggestion, working with children at the local shelter, was continuing to do what she loved.

Terri's gift—a white, fluffy doggie—went to Jacelyn. The stuffed animal, Terri explained, was a reminder that dogs and other pets were here to love and bless us, and to teach unconditional love. Her husband had talked her into accepting their dog Blue, and Terri most benefited from cuddling up with her during some of her darkest moments. Blue had become her baby and a true source of joy for the entire family.

Rainey opened Jolinda's gift of purple tulip bulbs. Jolinda revealed they were from her mother.

> She said, "Purple to me represents royalty. It's a deep, rich color of honor and beauty. When I think of spiritual growth, I think of nature and everything that grows. God's loving hand on us all nurturing, watering, and tending to us." Turning to Rainey, she said, "As you tend to the bulbs, planting, watering and watching them bloom, think of yourself and God watering your garden of life."

Opening the last gift, Terri received a coffee mug with the message, "Here's to strong women. May we know them, may we be them, may we raise them." That one needed no explanation!

After we all took a moment to breathe and laugh, I gave out my gift, the same to all. My message on their cards said: "I'm glad we had this magical dance together. Love, Victoria," followed by a stanza from Lord of the Dance by Sydney Carter:

> "Dance, then, wherever you may be, I am the Lord of the dance, said he,
> And I'll lead you on wherever you may be,
> I'll lead you on in the dance, said he!"

The gift itself was a medallion with "Love Rising" inscribed on the front, and "The Magical Dance" on the back.

Once again, I, the crybaby, was choking back tears. For any licensed psychologists who are saying I crossed professional lines, I do not fall in that category of therapist. Instead, in addition to holding a B.S. in Psychology, I'm a trained minister. We're referred to as Stephen Ministers, and we walk alongside folks as they are hurting. Our job is to point to healing. Serving in that capacity, I learned years ago to go deep from my heart with the ones whom God brings across my path. That's what I do best. Through my experience, love is the best healing agent of all. When love is the missing piece, I supply it and guide them to find more.

Love Rising Movement

When we slow down, love, and listen to others, it's a magical dance: the dance of love! My reason for sharing how one of my special dinners unfolded is to encourage small groups of women over the world to birth the same kind of nurturing occasions. My vision is that women who love, listen, nurture, and care for others will join the Love Rising Movement. In my twenty-plus years as a counselor and minister, I can assure you that women want the following:

L - Loved
O - Observed
V - Valued
E - Embraced
R - Ready
I - Inspiring
S - Sheltering
I - Infallible (Certain to Succeed)
N - Next Big Thing
G - Groundbreaker

165

Loved: To Understand Love, We Must First Love Ourselves

Love is the key ingredient to healing. When you feel love, you are connecting to the True Self, and the True Self is perfect, without flaw. Consequently, the more you can see and appreciate the perfection of spirit in your life and in those of everyone around you, the more you will feel healed and deeply loved.

You may feel you are not deserving of love. This feeling is particularly prevalent among those who struggle with addiction. Those in recovery must not only believe they are worthy of being loved, but they must also be open to accepting love from those around them and giving love in return, if they are to be successful on their path to wellness.

After self-love, you can share the overflow of love with those around you.

Self-love is the most important love you can invite into your life. If you care for and love yourself, you can share love with others. After learning to love and appreciate yourself, you find that the love overflows, and that's what you share with those around you. Giving of your time expands your heart. No matter how difficult your own life may seem, there is always someone in need of your attention, unique talents, and energy. Volunteering for causes that are important to you, like those that benefit the homeless, the elderly, or animals, can help you feel fulfilled and connect you with others who are also working to improve the world.

I have many special stories from our work with homeless ladies. We take baskets of love into the streets of Atlanta and into heavily prostituted areas and strip clubs. One afternoon, when I was getting ready to take the baskets out around Christmas, my team gave me a gift—a beautiful cross necklace with tiny diamonds. So precious, and a gift for our charity's fifth anniversary, the cross had special meaning to me, yet I felt a nudge that I would be giving it away that night. Later, when I met with the team, I asked if it would be okay if I did that. I was torn and secretly hoping they would say no. Instead, they all jumped up and down, and enthusiastically supported my request.

That evening, as we went out with our baskets of love, we met a special lady, T. Although I interacted with many others, T continued to come up in my mind. I had put the cross necklace in a little box.

Giving it to her, I said, "I feel this has your name on it."

She jumped up from her seat in the strip club dressing room and hugged me so tightly, and then tears came flowing down her cheeks.

"I just spent my last penny on my three girls," she confided. "You know I'm a single mother. I thought, after buying the girls' Christmas, there will not be any Christmas for me this year. And look what God did! I spent all the money I had on the girls and now this."

I told T to remember how special and loved she was, especially as she wore the necklace.

"You are loved!" I affirmed.

Our hearts were overflowing with love that evening.

Saltwater Tip: You can never out-give God. He always gives back more love than you or I can contain.

By the way, I've received countless necklaces since then. When I'm prompted, I always pass them on.

Loving yourself and loving others is a delight. You will get addicted, too, so pass it on!

Observed: To Be Noticed and Perceived as Significant

When we've observed something or someone, the thing or person is something we've noticed or perceived and registered as being significant.

You and I long to feel significant in our lives, in our relationships, and in our careers. Let's give others what we long for. Be grateful and thankful to others and let them know how much you appreciate them. Gratitude and appreciation return to you like a boomerang, and the blessings are big.

Valued: Paying Attention to What Matters Most

Singer-songwriter Fionna Apple provides a beautiful example of paying attention to what matters. Having released her first album in seven years, she posted a handwritten note on Facebook, notifying fans that she couldn't go on tour. Her dog Janet was dying.

> "It's 6 p.m. on Friday," she shared, "and I'm writing to a few thousand friends I have not met yet. I am writing to ask them to change our plans and meet a little while later. Here's the thing. I have a dog Janet, and she's been ill for almost two years now, as a tumor has been idling in her chest, growing ever so slowly. She's almost 14 years old now. I got her when she was 4 months old. I was 21 then, an adult officially—and she was my child."

Apple went on to say that Janet had been her constant companion, unlike any other. She couldn't bear the thought of not being there as a source of love and comfort during Janet's passing.

Let's pay attention to the things that matter most! Let's value others.

Embrace: Physical Touch Is a Healing Agent

Hugging allows us to show love, forgiveness, gratitude, and so many more positive emotions. While emotionally satisfying, hugging also provides health benefits, including lowering high blood pressure.

You don't need to suffer with a weak heart to gain something big from a hug: happiness! Hugging releases serotonin and dopamine, which lift your mood. Hugs further increase levels of oxytocin, a hormone that triggers the bonding response and makes you feel calmer and less anxious. Hugging promotes longevity and a stronger immune system, and some studies suggest that it reduces symptoms of Alzheimer's disease.

Embrace hugging. If you don't have a human nearby to hug, cuddle with a dog or cat. My cousin has a cat that kneads her stomach when she cramps!

Ready: Get Ready for Action

As you have loved yourself and others, and you are fully nurturing yourself, you'll find it's time for action. Ladies, the need to express the changes you are going through in a tangible way is universal during this passage. Go with the flow and don't worry about what others think.

Some try a different hairstyle or buy new clothes. Others concentrate on their homes or dedicate themselves to getting fit. Many pick up an instrument or go back to college. All are signs of taking action, of turning power surges and energy outward. The alterations are often symbolic; they set the stage for change and prepare you and others for a new future and telling the world: Here I come. Get ready. Make room for a new me.

You will become a new me during this transformation process. Like the metamorphosis of the caterpillar, you'll receive your wings, so prepare to fly!

Inspiring: This Is Your Bright-Light Season. Be an Inspiration to the World Around You.

You may be saying, "Well, Victoria, I do not feel like an inspiration." Start by saying a simple prayer in the morning:

Dear God, please allow me to touch at least one person today.

Make it a practice to look for one small thing you can do each day to share the gift of grace with anyone. It could be as simple as smiling at someone you see at a store or the gym. Or, visit an elderly home with gifts; send an anonymous note to someone, acknowledging his or her unique gift or talent; purchase a dozen roses and give one each to a coworker, neighbor, post office clerk, and so on; or run an errand for someone without being asked. One of my neighbors cut another neighbor's grass while the latter took an unexpected trip. Instead of returning home to a jungle, the family drove up to a nicely cut yard. What an amazing surprise!

Bringing an unexpected gift to someone who could use a message of love will also bless you in a big way.

Bigger ways to give include adopting a family in your community and sending an anonymous gift once a month; spending some time each week tutoring a child; interacting with an older person, who probably has a story to share; volunteering at your local shelter; serving as a Big Brother or Big Sister for a child in need.

Taking it further, you could start a not-for-profit organization that raises money for a meaningful cause. By investing your time and energy in a specific project, you not only give yourself a chance to make your spiritual values a more tangible part of your life, but you also build strong, intimate bonds with others. These relationships will have a direct influence on generations to come. Be an inspiration! Shine your light bright!

Trust me. You already are an inspiration, so keep going.

Sheltered: Taking Care of Tender Hearts

Now is the time to fight for a cause. One of my favorite children's stories, *Horton Hears a Who!* by Dr. Seuss, features Horton, an elephant who hears some noise coming from a speck of dust. Instead of ignoring the sound, he pays attention and learns that the tiny beings of Whoville need Horton's help. The other animals think he's crazy until the citizens of Whoville unite to make enough noise, shouting, "We are here! We are here! We are here!"

Be a Horton. Defend the least, the lost, and the abused with your life and your love. Fight for justice and shelter the hurting, the least among us. When people scream, *we are here*, will you help them? This is the season to take a stand.

Infallible: Certain to Succeed

Many women live their dreams as they approach and pass fifty. Kathryn Bigelow provides a wonderful example. She directed some small action movies, including *Point Break*, before receiving international acclaim for *The Hurt Locker* in 2008. At fifty-seven, she won Academy Awards for Best Picture and Best Director. She has also become a spokesperson for gender discrimination, noting how women directors do not receive equal opportunity.

Be confident. Your age is not a deterrent; it's an advantage. Consider all the experience and wisdom you've gained!

Next Big Thing: You Are the Next Big Thing!

Own it and walk in it! Remember the classic line from the movie *Fried Green Tomatoes*: "We are older, and we have more insurance!" Go for the big dream! You are mature, you have wisdom, and it's time for you to rock it! Show us what you've got! We are waiting and cheering you on.

Saltwater Tip: You are the next big thing. Make it happen!

Groundbreaker: It's Time to Reinvent Yourself

When seeking an example of someone who reinvented herself later in life, you cannot overlook Julia Child. For three decades, from the 1960s into the 1980s, she removed the mystique of French cooking by demonstrating you didn't have to be a trained chef to prepare and savor the most spectacular gourmet dishes.

With a career that began in advertising, she worked for the U.S. Government during World War II. In 1948, Julia and her husband moved to Paris, where she fell in love with French cuisine. Inspired to take a cooking class, she surprised everyone by mastering the skills to collaborate on the book *Mastering the Art of French Cooking.* Julia was fifty by the time she appeared on her first cooking show in 1963.

Laura Ingalls Wilder, author of the *Little House on the Prairie* book series, grew up in log cabins. Born in 1867, she and her pioneer family settled in Wisconsin, Missouri, Kansas, Minnesota, and the Dakotas when such places were considered America's wilderness. She worked as a schoolteacher, but only briefly before marrying and raising her family. When her daughter urged her to submit a story for a children's literature contest, Laura revised a manuscript that had previously been rejected. She won, and her first book was published. Laura Ingalls Wilder was sixty-five years old.

If you need more inspiration, search online for successful women over fifty, and you'll find countless examples from every century.

The bottom line is that every woman wants to be loved, observed, valued, and embraced. By giving l-o-v-e, love encompasses your spirit, and that's when you become empowered to change the world. When your love cup is full, look out, world!

Inspiring, sheltering, infallible, and certain to succeed, you and I are the next big thinkers and groundbreakers. Let's empower one another, one lady at a time. Let's reach out in love to change the world. *What the World Needs Now Is Love* is not only the title to my favorite song, but it's a truthful statement!

What's next? Aren't you craving more? Join me, then, in the Love Rising Movement.

Join the Love Rising Movement

"Once the soul awakens, the search begins and you can never go back. From then on, you are inflamed with a special longing that will never again let you linger in the lowlands of complacency and partial fulfillment. The eternal makes you urgent. You are loath to let compromise or the threat of danger hold you back from striving toward the summit of fulfillment."
John O'Donohue

Is it a life crisis or a spiritual calling?

Many of us have experienced permanent change during this menopausal passage. Some changes are delightful; some are not so great. Quite a few have referred to this season as a mid-life crisis. Such crises come in the form of an affair, a divorce, severe job unhappiness, an empty nest, lifeless relationships, endless life dissatisfaction, or disappointment with the way life has gone. Ultimately, the midlife crisis comes at a moment when you've gathered enough wisdom to know that you're not going to live forever. Most people who experience midlife crises have spent their entire lives raising a family or working in a career. They haven't had the time, or capacity, to ask the important questions in life. Eventually, something triggers a common question: is this all there is?

For many, the passage into menopause is also like experiencing a spiritual awakening. It's the season to develop the deep longing to find your life purpose and connect with your soul. The craving marks the beginning of true love rising. You may find, however, that you don't know where to start, and no matter how hard you try, you may not seem to connect with your soul. People have referred to that feeling of being cut off as the "Dark Night of the Soul," which is also the name of a sixteenth-century poem. Women express to me that they simply feel lost.

You may notice a dissatisfaction, but not the usual day-to-day kind of discontent. It's a deep, internal disappointment—a gaping inner void that constantly reminds you that something is missing from your life, and something at a core level is lost. If you feel that way, the loss is likely that connection to your soul. Don't despair. Although the period of unhappiness, confusion, and longing may feel like a bad thing at first, it is the greatest blessing you could receive. The spiritual awakening process may seem like a harrowing

Hero Story

Margaret Cohen, now in her seventies, became a professional skier at the age of fifty, when she started working as an instructor. She had lost her hearing, but with the help of cochlear implants, Margaret could participate and interact with others. Her message is not to focus on minor issues but to take advantage of opportunities that bring happiness and purpose to your life.

experience, but its sole purpose is to initiate you into your spiritual journey. Your spiritual journey is the very path that leads you to total healing, empowerment, and fulfillment.

My vision is to have groups of women from all over the world acknowledging and experiencing the spiritual journey of Love Rising.

I'll conduct Love Rising master classes through which I'll share why and how the process happens, as well as how to retrieve, explore, and communicate with your soul. The process of soul work will help you to live a life infused with meaning, beauty, joy, and love. Above all, Love Rising provides an anchor and much needed direction to birth your dreams.

The Love Rising movement exits to empower you to be all that you can be—mind, body, soul and spirit. The following modules will enable you to map out your spiritual journey:

Spiritual Awakening – You'll discover the surprising part of yourself that's been yearning to break free.

Determining the Enlightened Path – You'll gain clarity about the right path for you, and clear steps to achieve your dreams.

Removing the Obstacles – You'll gain clarity about the right path for you with clear steps to overcoming your biggest obstacle to serenity and joy, and learn powerful techniques to stay in your joy every day.

Continuing the Upward Spiral – When you're living your dreams, what else do you dream about? You'll discover how to create ever-increasing levels of bliss, excitement, and serenity in your life.

Learn all about Love Rising Master Classes at FindingHeavenBook.com.

I look forward to hearing from you. Oh, I can see Love Rising all over the world!

Thank you for buying *Finding Heaven in the Midst of Hormonal Hell.*

Please accept my FREE GIFT: 19 Ways to Improve Your Relationships
Increase your passion. Gain and establish trust.
Enjoy the love you've always wanted.
GO TO FindingHeavenBook.com/pages/bonus.

Saltwater Tips

Chapter 2
Choice and personal care unlock a joyous menopause.

Do an inventory of spiritual, mental, physical and social. Are they balanced?

The 7 Habits of Highly Successful People by Stephen Covey

Chapter 3
Fasting promotes healing.

The Complete Guide to Fasting by Jason Fung and Jimmy Moore

Fasting by Jenetzen Franklin

Make-Ahead Paleo by Tammy Credicott

Bone Broth Diet by Kellyann Petrucci, MS, ND

The Mediterranean Diet for Every Day: 4 Weeks of Recipes and Meal Plans to Lose Weight by Callisto Media

Nitric Oxide at FindingHeavenBook.com or your local health store without soy

Chapter 4
Tapping or EFT

The Tapping Solution by Nick Ortner

Rhodiola lowers cortisol at FindingHeavenBook.com

Chapter 5
Five Steps to Forgiveness: Victoria's Master Class at FindingHeavenBook.com

Chapter 6
Enjoy the pleasure of life, treating your body well.

Natural Remedies: Pueraria mirifica, maca, black cohosh, ground golden flaxseed, chasteberry at FindingHeavenBook.com

Chapter 7
Victoria's Masterclass: The Sword and Torch and Allowing Compassion at FindingHeavenBook.com

Chapter 8
Take time to love and heal your inner child.

Vaginal atrophy cream at Amatalife.com

Vitamin D at FindingHeavenBook.com

Chapter 9
Assess emotional and hormonal needs.

Learn Self Love: Victoria's Master Class at
FindingHeavenBook.com

Find your tribe/Birth a movement: Masters Class at
FindingHeavenBook.com

The Wisdom of Menopause, Dr. Christiane Northrup

Chapter 10
Love sets the stage for the miraculous.

You are the next big thing.

Join the Love Rising Movement at
FindingHeavenBook.com

Thank You for Reading *Finding Heaven in the Midst of Hormonal Hell*.

Please Accept My FREE GIFT: 19 Ways to Improve Your Relationships
Increase Your Passion. Gain and Establish Trust.
Enjoy the Love You've Always Wanted.
GO TO FindingHeavenBook.com/pages/bonus

From the Heart of Victoria

Many years ago, I found myself in a very difficult place. Being raped at sixteen years of age and getting in with the wrong crowd, I was bankrupt. From drugs and poor life choices, I ended up homeless. I met an amazing woman of grace named Pam Younker, and I will forever be grateful to her. Pam and her family took me in, and loved, cherished, and adored me. Through my season with this precious family, I began to see myself as special, and I realized that something bigger than I had brought me to this place of love. The more I loved myself, the more I was able to give back. Importantly, I first had to feel the love. Through Pam's guidance and tender loving care, I realized a God of the Universe existed, and His grace had brought me thus far.

I found a place where I felt forever safe, forever accepted, forever held, completely loved, and always wanted. That place is with Jesus! No matter your social class, race, background, religion or anything else favorable or unfavorable in the eyes of men, you are a child of God. He desires and longs for you to come into His family.

All you have to say is, Jesus, remember me. He will come and take a place in your heart and fill your cup with the most irresistible love. As you fill up on His love, you will be a bright light in the world!

Let your lights shine brightly!

All of my love,

Victoria

$\mathcal{N}otes$

Chapter One: A Sticky Situation
Puleo, Stephen 2004
Dark Tide: The Great Boston Molasses Flood of 1919
Boston: Beacon Press.

Chapter Two: Life Is Like a Jigsaw Puzzle
Leaf, Caroline, Dr. 2013
Switch on your Brain: The Key to Peak Happiness Thinking and Health
Michigan: Baker Books

Northrup, Christiane M.D. 2006
The Wisdom of Menopause
New York: Bantam

Taub, Edward A, M.D., F.A.A.P. and Ferid, Murad F.A.A.P. and Oliphant, David M.D. 2007.,
The Wellness Solution
New York: Simon & Schuster Inc

Chapter Three: French Fry or Die! Give Me Those Fries!
Axe, Josh DNM, DC, CNS (2018), January 8
7 Benefits of Fasting + the Best Types of Fasting
Retrieved from https://draxe.com/benefits-fasting/

Chapter Four: Crashing Down
Ortner, Nick 2013
The Tapping solution: A Revolutionary System for Stress Free Living
United States: Hay House

Wells, Zoe N.D 2013
Women's Transformational Journey - 5 Steps to Creating Joy and Balance in Perimenopause
California: Zoe Wells Publishing

Chapter Five: Overcoming Gossip and Cliques
Neuharth, Dan, Ph.D.,(2017), August 9
Narcissim Decoded, *"Psyche Central,"*
Retrieved from https://blogs.psychcentral.com/narcissism-decoded/about/

Ortner, Jessica 2018, February 10
Judgement Detox: How to Eliminate the Energetic Drain of Judgement
From Your Life Force with Gabby Bernstein
Retrieved from https://thetappingsolution.com/2018tws/

Chapter Six: Stand Strong, Hold Your Ground
Ferguson, A. S. "Plato's Simile of Light. (Part II.) The Allegory of the Cave (Continued)". The Classical Quarterly 16, no. 1 (1922): 15–28.

Ortner, Jessica 2018, February 10
Who do you Think you are? How to Make Little Shifts in your Identity to Radically Transform your Future with Brad Yates.
Retrieved from https://thetappingsolution.com/2018tws/

Chapter Eight: It's Hot? Oh, Yeah, Sizzling Hot
Borchard, T. (2015). 6 Steps to Help Heal Your Inner Child. *Psych Central.*
Retreived from https://psychcentral.com/blo g/6-steps-to-help-heal-your-inner-child/

Bachman. G. (2016) February 17 Vaginal Atrophy
Retrieved from:https://www.mayoclinic.org/ diseases-conditions/vaginal-atrophy/symptoms-causes/ syc-20352288

Jaroenporn, Sukanya, (2014). "Improvements of Vaginal Atrophy Without Systemic Side Effects after Topical Application of Pueraria mirifica, a Phytoestrogen-rich Herb, in Postmenopausal Cynomolgus Macaques," *Journal of Reproduction and Development* 60, no. 3: 238– 454.

Chapter Nine: Finding What Works for You
Calabrese, J. HMC, CCH (2001) January Homeopathic Medicine for the Millennial
Retrieved from: http://www.homeopathyforwomen.org/ menopause.htm

Chang, L. (2015). "Americans Spend an Alarming Amount of Time Checking Social Media on Their Phones."
Retrieved from: http://www.digitaltrends.com/mobile/ informate-report-social-media-smartphone-use/

Made in the USA
Columbia, SC
03 November 2018